INTERNATIONAL SERIES IN
EXPERIMENTAL PSYCHOLOGY
GENERAL EDITOR: H. J. EYSENCK

VOLUME 20

AFFECT AND MEMORY
A REFORMULATION

OTHER TITLES IN THE SERIES IN EXPERIMENTAL PSYCHOLOGY

Vol. 1 Gray: *Pavlov's Typology*
Vol. 2 Holland: *The Spiral After-effect*
Vol. 3 Lynn: *Attention, Arousal and the Orientation Reaction*
Vol. 4 Claridge: *Personality and Arousal*
Vol. 5 Fellows: *The Discrimination Process and Development*
Vol. 6 Beech and Fransella: *Research and Experiment in Stuttering*
Vol. 7 Joffe: *Prenatal Determinants of Behaviour*
Vol. 8 Martin and Levey: *The Genesis of the Classical Conditioned Response*
Vol. 9 Baird: *Psychophysical Analysis of Visual Space*
Vol. 10 Meldman: *Diseases of Attention and Perception*
Vol. 11 Shaw and Sichel: *Accident Proneness*
Vol. 12 Lynn: *Personality and National Character*
Vol. 13 Feldman and McCulloch: *Homosexual Behaviour: Therapy and Assessment*
Vol. 14 Stroh: *Vigilance*
Vol. 15 Rachman: *Effects of Psychotherapy*
Vol. 16 Kolers: *Effects of Motion Perception*
Vol. 17 Levi: *Stress and Distress in Response to Psychological Stimuli*
Vol. 18 Claridge: *Personality Differences and Biological Variations: A Study of Twins*
Vol. 19 Frank: *Psychiatric Diagnosis: A Review of Research*

AFFECT AND MEMORY
A REFORMULATION

by

SATRAJIT DUTTA

Psychology Department, University of New Brunswick,
Fredericton, New Brunswick

and

RABINDRA NATH KANUNGO

Faculty of Management, McGill University, Montreal

PERGAMON PRESS

OXFORD • NEW YORK • TORONTO
SYDNEY • PARIS • BRAUNSCHWEIG

U.K.	Pergamon Press Ltd., Headington Hill Hall, Oxford OX3 0BW, England
U.S.A.	Pergamon Press Inc., Maxwell House, Fairview Park, Elmsford, New York 10523, U.S.A.
CANADA	Pergamon of Canada, Ltd., 207 Queen's Quay West, Toronto 1, Canada
AUSTRALIA	Pergamon Press (Aust.) Pty. Ltd., 19a Boundary Street, Rushcutters Bay, N.S.W. 2011, Australia
FRANCE	Pergamon Press SARL, 24 rue des Ecoles, 75240 Paris, Cedex 05, France
WEST GERMANY	Pergamon Press GMbH, 3300 Braunschweig, Postfach 2923, Burgplatz 1, West Germany

First edition 1975

Library of Congress Cataloging in Publication Data

Dutta, Satrajit.
Affect and memory: a reformulation.
(International series in experimental psychology; v 20)
Includes bibliographical references and index.
1. Affect (Psychology) 2. Memory.
I. Kanungo, Rabindra Nath, joint author.
II. Title. [DNLM: 1. Affect. 2. Memory.
BF511 D979a]
BF511.D85 1975 153.1'2 75–8628
ISBN 0 08 018270 4

Typesetting by Express Litho Service (Oxford)
Printed in Great Britain by A. Wheaton & Co. Exeter

Contents

Preface

The relationship between affect and memory as an issue has a history older than the discipline of psychology itself. Philosophers like Nietzsche and Schopenhauer had speculated on the dynamics of affect–memory relationship long before psychology was recognized as an experimental science. From the time psychology became an independent science, the issue has been one of the main concerns of experimental, social, and clinical psychologists. Its long history has produced a dense jungle of theories, explanations, and empirical findings. Several years ago, out of curiosity, we ventured to travel through this jungle and on our way we found ourselves totally lost. This book is the product of our desire to find our way out of the jungle. It presents the route we have taken in the form of a conceptual framework. The framework seems to explain and integrate apparently diverse and often contradictory theories and empirical findings in the area. We are not sure how far the path we are treading can lead us. Whatever distance we have moved along this path only gives us a sense of optimism. Through a series of experiments reported in this book we have attempted to demonstrate the usefulness of the framework for developing a better understanding of affect–memory relationship and for giving some direction to future research in that area.

At various stages of our work we have benefited from the interest and critical comments of many colleagues. We are indebted to all of them. In particular, we would like to thank William Caird, James Clark, and Bruce Earhard of Dalhousie University; Wallace Lambert and Alex Whitmore of McGill University; and Allen Paivio of the University of Western Ontario for their comments and suggestions on one or more parts of the manuscript.

Preparation of the manuscript was very much facilitated by technical assistance from Richard Gurekas, Clara Wong, and Anne Martin, and by nontechnical support and understanding from Minati Kanungo. It is a pleasure to record our gratitude to each of them.

Finally, we wish to thank the American Psychological Association for permission to reproduce materials from the *Journal of Personality and Social Psychology*.

Satrajit Dutta
Rabindra N. Kanungo

CHAPTER 1

Introduction

The Importance of Affect in Memory

Human memory is selective. We tend to remember better some of our experiences than others. Why we remember some experiences better than others is a question that has been a serious concern of psychologists for more than half a century. In attempting to answer the question, Freud (1925) proposed that the affect attached to our personal experiences is a major variable that determines selectivity in human memory. According to Freud, experiences associated with unpleasant affect are forgotten more rapidly than experiences associated with either pleasant or neutral affect. From the time of Freud's writings, the functional relationship between selective memory and affect of personal experiences has been considered to be of basic theoretical significance to general principles of learning and forgetting. Attempts at understanding the relationship have been a concern not only of psychologists interested in clinical problems (Alper, 1952; Eriksen, 1954; Freud, 1925; Rapaport, 1959; Rosenzweig, 1943) but also of experimental psychologists interested in learning and memory processes (McGeoch and Irion, 1952; Osgood, 1953; Weiner, 1966a, b) and social psychologists interested in social motivation and interpersonal and intergroup behavior (Atkinson, 1953; Edwards, 1942; Kanungo and Das, 1960; Taft, 1954). Clinical psychologists have viewed the phenomenon of selective memory for affective experiences as a form of ego defense or as mechanisms of personal adjustment. Experimental psychologists have tried to look for stimulus characteristics such as affective quality or affective intensity to explain the phenomenon. Social psychologists have emphasized the role of attitudes as mediating variables while dealing with the phenomenon. Thus one finds a wide range of interest among psychologists who tend to research the problem with a wide variety of research techniques. Despite the diversity of research conducted in this area, the efforts of various investigators over the last five decades or so, as reviewed in the next chapter, have resulted in a host of ambiguous and conflicting reports. Moreover, the results reported in most of the earlier studies appear to be inconclusive, difficult to interpret, and generally of dubious validity.

Stages in Memory Process and Limitations of Early Research

The most common confusion manifested in the earlier studies is their failure to distinguish, both conceptually and operationally, between different phases in the memory process which is suggested to be a multi-stage mechanism by various researchers (e.g., Cameron, 1947; Melton, 1963; Rapaport, 1959). The initial phase of memory process refers to sensory or ideational registration of a stimulus item as well as the fixation of the memory trace. This is the stage of learning, acquisition, or trace formation. The second phase involves a temporal interval between trace formation and trace retrieval during which the trace is latent but potentially available for retrieval. This phase is defined as the period of retention or trace storage. During this phase several dynamic and autonomous processes have been suggested to be operative to influence the memory traces, e.g., perseveration and consolidation (Glickman, 1961; Muller and Pilzecker, 1900; Walker, 1958); autonomous decay (Brown, 1958; Koffka, 1935); reverberation (Hebb, 1949), and integration and organization (Bartlett, 1932; Koffka, 1935). Other mechanisms through which additional informational inputs can modify or alter the memory traces during the storage phase are suggested to be unlearning (Barnes and Underwood, 1959; Briggs, 1954; Melton and Irwin, 1940) and interference (McGeoch, 1932; Postman, 1961; Underwood, 1957). The third and final stage in the memory sequence is the recall phase which involves trace evocation or retrieval. At this stage even a potentially available item may not be accessible due to repression (Freud, 1925) or some interference mechanisms (Holmes and Schallow, 1969).

Thus inaccessibility of a memory item at the time of recall may be either due to its inadequate or poor registration in the first place or due to weakening or wiping out of the trace during storage phase, or even due to the possibility that a potentially available trace is prevented from being recalled by some interference mechanism. It is thus obvious that manipulation of affective variables at any of these three phases in the multi-stage sequential process of memory can conceivably affect or influence recall. Yet, in almost all the studies in this area, manipulations of affective variables have been employed at the time of stimulus registration, and hardly any attempt has been made to study the effect of manipulation of affect either on the storage or on the retrieval mechanism. It is to be noted in this connection that despite the conceptual distinction between storage and retrieval it is found extremely difficult, if not impossible, to distinguish between these two phases of memory in operational terms. That is, any effect of an affective variable, introduced following registration, on recall may be attributed to changes produced either in the storage or in the retrieval mechanism. But to isolate one effect from another and make conclusive inferences regarding such effects as separate from and independent of each other is made difficult by the fact that recall as a measure refers merely to the accessibility of items and not to their availability.

Furthermore, as noted already, the studies in this area have generally produced highly inconsistent and inconclusive results. There were several methodological difficulties faced by the investigators which at least partially account for the inconsistency of their results. Firstly, in experiments designed to study the effect of affective tone of items on their memory value, it proved difficult to isolate the variable of affect from other potent variables influencing learning and forgetting, such as frequency, familiarity, motivational relevance, meaningfulness, recency, rehearsal, and so on. Secondly, it has proven equally difficult to specify the exact extent and nature of the affective properties of the material learned. Inadequate control of either the quality or the intensity of the feeling tone of the memory items as perceived by the subjects in many cases gave rise to ambiguous results that were difficult to interpret. Lack of an integrative approach to the problem in theoretical terms as well as procedural variations from one study to another have merely added to the confusion.

Finally, most of the studies in this area were reported during the first half of this century. As Weiner (1966b) observes, there has been very little additional literature in this area since the 1940s, although the basic problem concerning the role of affect in memory remains essentially unsolved. When viewed in terms of the present-day context of methodological rigor and sophistication, many of the earlier studies are characterized by questionable method, poor design, and arbitrary procedural technique. A more detailed review of the studies will be presented in Chapter 2.

Some recent studies in the area of selective retention of affective material (Dutta and Kanungo, 1967; Dutta *et al.*, 1972; Kanungo, 1968; Kanungo and Dutta, 1966) have suggested that the intensity, rather than the quality, of perceived affect of experiences influences their selective retention. The intensity hypothesis proposed by these investigators specifies the functional relationship between affectivity and retention in terms of perceived intensity of affect. According to this hypothesis, the perceived intensity of an affective experience varies with the degree of an individual's emotional involvement in a situation. It is suggested that any variable that can bring about changes in perceived intensity of affective experiences is also a variable that indirectly influences their selective retention because, in the ultimate analysis, the more intense the perceptual affectivity of an experience, the better is its retention. Thus it is proposed that a comprehensive theoretical model, in terms of affective intensity, may be found quite adequate to explain most of the research findings in the area of selective retention of affective experiences.

General Plan of the Book

To present a comprehensive account of the intensity hypothesis, to review and evaluate the findings reported in the studies mentioned above as verification of the hypothesis, and to critically examine the implications of such findings for an integrative theoretical model are the primary objectives that essentially define the plan of this book. The sequence and organization of the chapters inevitably reflect the ways in which research in the area has proceeded in the past several years. In Chapter 2 an attempt is made to orient the reader to the problem of the role of affect in memory. Consequently the chapter puts the problem in a historical perspective and critically reviews the existing literature from methodological and theoretical standpoints. Following this general orientation and review, in Chapter 3 the main characteristics of "the intensity of perceived affect hypothesis" is proposed, and a comparative account of the hypothesis as opposed to earlier versions of stimulus intensity hypothesis is presented. Chapters 4 and 5 describe empirical studies that provide evidence on the role of intensity of perceived affect in selective memory. The effects of intensity of perceived affect on learning are dealt with in the same chapters; its effects on retrieval process are considered. In Chapter 6 an attempt is made to propose an integrative framework that explains the diverse findings stemming from contemporary work, and points the way toward future directions which might be taken in experimental research in the area of affect and selective memory. Finally, the same chapter includes a brief discussion of the practical implications of the research findings in the area of attitude change, communication, and interpersonal relations.

CHAPTER 2

Historical Retrospect

Origin and Perspective of the Inquiry

An early analytic and fairly systematic attempt to ascertain the relationship between perceived affect and selective retention was made by Bartlett (1932). Bartlett emphasized the influence of emotional attitude on the memorization of everyday experiences, and pointed out that one's emotional attitude tended to influence and transform the nature of any event stored in memory at the time of recall or reproduction. Any survey of the experimental research addressed to the problem should, however, refer to studies conducted much earlier than 1932, the year of the publication of Bartlett's book *Remembering.* In such a historical review, Colgrove's (Rapaport, 1959, p. 43) questionnaire study in 1899 may be mentioned as the first empirical approach to the problem. Since then numerous studies concerned in various ways with the relation of memory to affective processes have been conducted. Rapaport (1959) made a systematic analysis of diverse viewpoints and research findings in this area. For comprehensive surveys of most of the studies reported before the forties, Barrett (1938), Cason (1932), Gilbert (1938), Jersild (1931), Meltzer (1930), and Moore (1935) may be consulted. Reviews of more recent studies can be found in Dudycha and Dudycha (1941), Edwards (1942), Goldin (1964), McGeoch and Irion (1952), Osgood (1953), Weiner (1966a), and Zeller (1952).

Most of the early and many of the recent studies have been attempts to test an implication of the Freudian theory of repression. It is to be noted at the outset that the theory of repression (just as most of the subsequent theories related to the problem and reviewed later in this chapter) considered affective *quality* rather than *quantity* or intensity as the crucial determinant of selective retention of affective experiences. When reduced to the simplified form, the repression theory assumes that pleasant experiences are remembered better than unpleasant experiences.† The contention that forgotten experiences are mostly those which are unpleasant, anxiety-provoking, or painful to an individual, was derived from clinical case studies. Freud's

†A more adequate description of Freud's concept of repression is given on p.11.

pioneering work in this area stimulated the enthusiasm of the later researchers who engaged themselves in experimental investigation of the problem. This has resulted in a large number of laboratory studies which provide a relevant and wide background against which different facets of the problem can be studied and evaluated.

Rapaport (1959) points out that in addition to Freud's book *On the Psychopathology of Everyday Life* (1914) there were two other factors which contributed to the active interest and orientation assumed by investigators inquiring into the relationship between quality of feeling tone and selective memory. First, the *fin-de-siècle* mood and the pessimistic philosophy of Schopenhauer had an overwhelming influence on humanistic science in general. The age-old debate regarding the essential optimism or pessimism of human beings reached almost a crescendo at this time and inspired numerous investigators in the field of memory to pursue the problem of whether pleasant or unpleasant experiences were better remembered.

The second influence affecting theories in this area was the pleasure–pain theory of learning. Originated by Bain (1868) and Spencer (1873), this hedonistic theory exerted great influence on latter-day education psychology and specifically on Thorndike's (1923, 1927) "law of effect" which stated that a satisfying consequence "stamped in" an experience and one followed by an annoying state is "stamped out".

The research on this hedonistic position started with the assumption that the retention of pleasant (P) material was greater than unpleasant (U) material. The body of research produced by such investigations is extremely inconclusive. In some cases, U recall was found to be less than P recall (Jersild, 1931; Meltzer, 1930; Stagner, 1931, for example); in others, the results failed to confirm the above findings (cf. Menzies, 1935; Waters and Leeper, 1936), and even mixed results were obtained within the same experiment (Thompson, 1930).

Methodological Considerations

In view of the procedural diversity of these studies, McGeoch and Irion (1952) suggested three major categories in terms of which the experimental investigations could be broadly classified.

A. *The Method of Free Recall*

This category includes those studies which used the method of free recall of experiences of everyday life. Subjects were instructed to recall all of their experience during a specified period of time. They were also asked to rate these experiences as pleasant (P), unpleasant (U), and neutral (N). The degree of the difference between P and U experiences recalled was considered as the criterion of inference as to which experiences had greater retention value. Some of the representative studies in this category were reported by Henderson (1911), Jersild (1931), Koch (1930), O'Kelley and Steckle (1940), Stagner (1931), Thomson (1930), Waters and Leeper (1936), and Wohlgemuth (1923).

Meltzer (1930) asserted that only this method of recalling everyday life experiences was a valid and realistic method by which selective retention of P and U experiences could be studied. According to Meltzer, use of materials not relevant to subjects' interests and artificial conditions of the laboratory make other procedures inapplicable to the study of feeling responses and their selective retention in real life situations. Edwards (1942) shared the view championed by Meltzer. After reviewing the studies conducted following this method, the main findings were summarized by Edwards (p. 45) as follows:

> First, at the initial recall period a predominant number of pleasant experiences are reported. Second, at subsequent recall periods both extremely pleasant and unpleasant experiences tend to be remembered better than those which are neutral. Third, of the two extremes (pleasant and unpleasant) the pleasant experiences tend to be remembered better than the unpleasant.

The interpretation of these findings is made difficult by ambiguities in the method of free recall. Rapaport (1959) raised certain doubts regarding the validity of this method though he recognized the greater personal relevance of life experiences as opposed, for instance, to arbitrarily selected P and U words or P and U sensory material. He questioned whether subjects would communicate their relevant emotional experiences to the experimenter. He also expressed doubt whether affectively toned experiences could be adequately verbalized by the average subjects. McGeoch and Irion (1952) considered the method of free recall to be unreliable because the results might be influenced by several unknown variables such as temporary set, self-instruction on the part of subjects, and the relative frequencies of the occurrence of P and U experience. It was also proposed by McGeoch and Irion that the results would be influenced by whether the experiences were rated by subjects in terms of their original affective value or on the basis of the affective value of those experiences as perceived by them at the time of rating. Furthermore it was noted that the recall of more experiences rated pleasant than unpleasant might reflect a favorable disposition of subjects toward past events of their lives (Barrett, 1938; Cason, 1932). Finally, according to Osgood (1953), selective rehearsal of the highly pleasant experiences during the retention interval might inflate the recall of subjects in favor of P experiences. Obviously, in that case, the obtained results merely indicated frequent practice of the pleasant rather than a stronger memory value for the pleasant.

Thus the lack of control of a number of variables as described above makes the results of the experiences using the method of free recall "... too complicated to interpret confidently" (McGeoch and Irion 1952, p. 385).

B. *The Method of Affective Pairing*

The second widely used procedure to investigate retention of affective material is that of affective pairing. This procedure involves the pairing of affectively toned sensory experience with a relatively indifferent or neutral verbal symbol such as nonsense syllable or number. The assumption is that the symbols will take on the affective value of the experiences with which they have been paired. Any influence of affective tone on memory should thus be revealed in a subsequent attempt to recall the symbols. Ratliff's (1938) representative study using this method may be mentioned in this connection. In Ratliff's study, lists of numbers paired with sensory items, such as sounds, colors, and odors, evaluated in terms of pleasantness and unpleasantness, were presented to subjects. Results revealed that although the differences between the recall of numbers in response to P and U stimuli were in no case significant, recall was uniformly better and the reaction time faster in the case of numbers which had been paired with P sound and color stimuli than in the case of numbers paired with U sound and color stimuli. In the case of olfactory stimuli, however, opposite results were obtained. Other studies have followed a method slightly different from that used by Ratliff. In these studies unpleasant or disturbing sensory impressions are interpolated into the process of memorization of indifferent verbal material (Frank and Ludwigh, 1931; Harden, 1930; Stone, 1925). The results of at least two of these studies have proven to be inconclusive. Frank and Ludwigh, however, did find that recall was facilitated by interpolated P odors, whereas interpolated U odors inhibited recall. In a subsequent experiment, Frank (1931) attempted to find out whether the facilitating effect of P odors as observed in the earlier study was due to the affective tones associated with them or was attributable to the odors themselves. The results obtained by him seemed to confirm the latter hypothesis.

While the method of affective pairing does not share with the method of free recall such deficiencies as an uncontrolled frequency of P and U items, the former method is based on the unverified presumption that neutral items take on the feeling tone of affective materials with which they are paired. Moreover, because of the inconsistent results obtained, the studies reported using this method failed to make any conclusive statement regarding perceived affect of materials and their selective retention.

C. *The Method of Retention of Affectively Toned Items*

The third and most widely used traditional method of examining the retention of affectively toned items uses a list of verbal or non-verbal items which are evaluated as P, U, and N by subjects. Subjects are later asked to recall, rehearse, or recognize these items. In some of the earlier experiments the affective tone of the items was determined either by the experimenter (studies by Tait as well as Tolman, cited by Rapaport, 1959, p. 79), by judges not included in the experimental group (Chaney and Lauer, 1929), or by having the words first rated by the experimental group on the basis of which the final selection of the words was made (e.g., Carter and Jones, 1937; White and Powell, 1936; White and Ratliff, 1934). In some other studies (Fox, 1923, for example), materials, such as names of people and objects, portraits, picture postcards, etc., were used, and subjects were asked to evaluate these items in terms of like and dislike. More recently, Amster (1964) attempted to relate the subjective evaluation of words in terms of "good" or "bad" feeling tone associated with them to selective recall.

In a summary of the results of the experiments which compared the recall of words of different affective ratings, McGeoch and Irion (1952) have noted that the majority of the experiments show that retention tends to decrease in the order of P-U-N. They also note that the observed differences have been small, and there are many instances of contradictory results.

This procedure, like the previous procedures described, is deficient in a number of respects. McGeoch and Irion (1952) described two of these deficiencies. There is no evidence that items judged in isolation to have certain affective characteristics retain the same intensity and quality of feeling tone when combined with other items in lists or pairs. Nor is it necessarily the case that items will retain their initial tone during successive presentations. Since the data presented by Beebe-Centre (1932) on affective habituation seem to support this suspicion, it is difficult to disregard the relevance of McGeoch's and Irion's criticism.

Because of the methodological inadequacies and inconsistent results as mentioned above, the studies using this method did not prove to be any more satisfactory than those discussed earlier.

In general, the studies in this area, regardless of the methods used, have offered very little in the way of straightforward conclusions. Moreover, the methodological deficiencies discussed above have provided fertile soil for theoretical controversies to flourish.

Theoretical Considerations

Historically speaking, Freud's translation of traditional hedonistic notions into his theory of repression was the first theoretical attempt to establish a functional relationship between memory and affective experiences. In view of the inadequacies of the Freudian theory, several other alternative theories and explanatory principles have subsequently been suggested by different investigators. It is to be noted that all but one of these theoretical positions essentially emphasize the nature or quality of affect as the crucial predictor of selective memory. In contrast to these qualitative approaches, the intensity or quantitative approach discussed in detail in Chapter 3 considers perceived intensity or magnitude of feeling tone as the crucial variable which more adequately predicts selective retention. While qualitative positions generally place emphasis on the quality of feeling tone as the determinant of selective retention, they differ from each other only insofar as their respective points of emphasis refer to different aspects or attributes of the affective quality of experiences and different mechanisms underlying these experiences. Five major qualitative positions will be reviewed in this chapter, followed by a discussion of the quantitative approach in Chapter 3. It should be pointed out that the five qualitative positions discussed are not mutually exclusive; on the contrary, both conceptually and methodologically they very much overlap. Yet insofar as it is possible to distinguish between certain major theoretical trends, distinctive orientations, or points of emphasis, a workable classificatory scheme is warranted.

The theoretical positions of qualitative approaches may be classified as follows:

(a) The *hedonistic* position which suggests, mostly in terms of the concept of repression, that pleasant experiences are retained better than unpleasant experiences.
(b) The *tension system* position, which emphasizes concepts such as unresolved tension systems or closure felt in connection with an experience as the crucial variables in terms of which selective retention of the experience can be explained.

(c) The *personality type* or differential position, which attempts to explain different patterns of selective retention of pleasant and unpleasant experiences in terms of different personality orientations or dispositions that tune individuals to emphasize on either ego-threatening or ego-enhancing aspects of their experiences.

(d) The *contextual* position, which suggests that fittingness of experiences with the existing mental set, context, or frame of reference of individuals is the crucial variable in terms of which conflicting experimental findings in this area can be explained.

(e) The *retroactive inhibition* position, which attempts to explain the general superiority of pleasant over unpleasant recall in terms of the classical concept of retroactive inhibition or interference.

A. *The Hedonistic Position*

According to the pleasure principle implied by classical hedonism, any organism is assumed to seek pleasure and avoid displeasure. The Freudian version of this pleasure principle, as reflected in his hypothesis of repression (1925), suggests that forgetting of unpleasant experiences may be explained by a tendency on the part of an individual to avoid painful and anxiety-provoking memories. It is proposed by Freud that in order to avoid pain and anxiety, unpleasant experiences are pushed below the threshold of consciousness through the defense mechanism of repression.

Some of those who have attempted to test the repression hypothesis have assumed that a sufficient condition for the operation of repression is the occurrence of an unpleasant experience. Others (Goldin, 1964; McGranahan, 1940; Rosenzweig, 1938; Sears, 1936) have pointed out that for the initiation of a defensive control the self-esteem or conscience of an individual must come into conflict with some positive drive on his part. As noted by Goldin (1964), it is uncertain whether Freud himself clearly distinguished between repression of anxiety-provoking experience and defensive reaction against any form of unpleasant stimuli. It has been clearly shown by Madison (1961) that Freud used repression to refer to the general process of defense throughout his writings. In any case, on the basis of the revision of the original psychoanalytic concept of repression, as proposed by Goldin (1964) and others, most of the investigations of the recall of P and U experiences, reviewed earlier, cannot be regarded as adequate tests of the strict Freudian repression hypothesis.

The studies which attempted to test the general hedonistic proposition that P recall was superior to U recall, not necessarily in terms of the concept of repression, failed to produce any definite conclusion. Apart from the methodological inadequacies discussed earlier, the results generated by them were highly contradictory and inconclusive. There were numerous studies (e.g., Balken, 1933; Cason and Lungren, 1932; Chaney and Lauer, 1929; Menzies, 1935; Silverman and Cason, 1934; Waters and Leeper, 1936; Wohlgemuth, 1923) which either failed to show any superiority of P over U recall or produced contrary results.

More recently, several attempts have been reported to test the strict Freudian repression hypothesis (Aborn, 1953; Flavell, 1955; Merrill, 1954; Penn, 1964; Truax, 1957; Weiner, 1968; Zeller, 1950b, 1952). Most of these studies follow an experimental research paradigm developed by Zeller (1950a) for empirical tests of the repression concept. The paradigm involves three phases. In the first phase, both experimental and control subjects learn and recall a list of words. In the second phase, the experimental subjects undergo an ego-threatening experience, while the control subjects are not exposed to any threatening experience. After the threat manipulation, a second recall test is given. Since it is assumed that anxiety caused by threat will generalize to words learned in the same laboratory situation, and since it is also assumed that anxiety is painful and results in repression, it is predicted that in the second recall test experimental subjects will perform below the level of control subjects. In the third phase, through experimental manipulation, the threat is eliminated, and consequently the repression is lifted and a third test is given. It is predicted that there will be no difference in recall between the groups in the third test. The studies following the paradigm have generally found experimentally induced repression to be effective in influencing selective memory. The relevance and significance of these studies, however, to the general problem of how P and U experiences are functionally related to the process of selective retention are quite restricted. For example, recently D'Zurilla (1965) and Holmes (1972), using similar experimental paradigm described above, have obtained results that question the validity of the repression interpretation of selective memory. In a post-experimental interview, D'Zurilla (1965) found that 62% of experimental subjects engaged in thoughts related to their threat experiences. This was contrary to what would be expected on the basis of repression explanation. One might argue that perhaps the threatening experiences for the experimental subjects in D'Zurilla's study were not intense enough to make the subjects use repression as their defense. If this argument be accepted as a valid one, then one must agree with Holmes's (1972) conclusion that "Zeller's (1950a) paradigm cannot be used to provide evidence for the concept of repression. This leaves the concept of repression in a precarious position with respect to the necessary experimental verification" (p. 170).

B. *The "Tension System" Position*

Zeigarnik (1938) was the first investigator to use the interrupted task technique in order to study the effect of interruption of an ongoing task on selective memory. She presented a number of tasks to subjects who were allowed to finish one half of the tasks. The remaining tasks were interrupted before completion. It was found that interrupted tasks were more often recalled than completed tasks. This phenomenon, popularly known as the Zeigarnik effect, was explained in terms of the concept of unresolved "tension systems" formulated by Lewin (1935). Tension systems were described by Lewin as forces generated by some psychological needs and quasi-needs in the psychological life space of an individual. Such tensions were suggested as determining the observed tendency on the part of an individual to resume or to perseverate in an interrupted activity. This observation, corroborated by many other investigators (Harrower, 1932, for example), is also considered as a confirmation of the well-known Gestalt principle of "closure". Nowlis (1941) and others have attributed the Zeigarnik effect to subjects' feelings of failure or success when their tasks were interrupted or not interrupted before completion. Marrow (1938a) found that when subjects were made to believe that interruption meant a successful performance and completion a poor performance, the Zeigarnik effect was reversed; subjects more frequently recalled the uninterrupted tasks. Presumably, successful completion of a task is perceived by an individual as pleasant, and incompletion as unpleasant. It could thus be concluded on the basis of the results of Zeigarnik's study that unpleasant tasks are recalled better than pleasant tasks in this particular experimental context.

Studies concerned with the effect of unresolved tension due to interruption on memory (Baddeley, 1963; Bogulavsky and Gutherie, 1941; Marrow, 1938a, b; Nowlis, 1941; Pachauri, 1935; Prentice, 1943) were, however, no less conflicting in their results than those representing the hedonistic positions discussed earlier. Lack of adequate control of a number of variables, such as degree of motivational involvement, task duration, recall interval, etc., may account for the inconsistency of their results.

Rosenzweig suggested, on the basis of results obtained in a series of experiments (1933a, b, 1936, 1938, 1941, 1943), that the Zeigarnik effect directly varied with the strength of motivation on the part of subjects toward the tasks. He further proposed that, in case of high motivational involvement, completed tasks would be recalled more frequently. Rosenzweig (1941, 1943) hypothesized two types of reaction tendencies, namely, need-persistive and ego-defensive. According to him, under conditions of low motivational stress induced by the experimental context (mild experience of failure), need-persistive reactions would predominate, whereas, under high stress condition produced by ego-threatening situation (intense experience of failure), ego-defensive reactions would become stronger. Although the results obtained by him under a low stress condition were similar to Zeigarnik's effect, the results were reversed under a high stress condition. Glixman (1949) introduced three levels or degrees of stress and results reported by him supported Rosenzweig's contention. Lewis (Lewis, 1944; Lewis and Franklin, 1944) also obtained results consistent with Rosenzweig's findings. However, several other investigators have failed to find any consistent effects of degree of experimentally induced stress on the selective recall of completed and incompleted tasks when subjects were unselected for personality variables (Alper, 1946a, b, 1957; Atkinson, 1953; Atkinson and Raphelson, 1956; Caron and Wallach, 1957; Eriksen, 1954).

It was noted by McGeoch and Irion (1952) that even when the differences were found in the direction predicted on the basis of the classical Zeigarnik effect, such differences were seldom very large. McGeoch and Irion further suggested the possibility that interruption, in certain cases, might have caused the interrupted tasks to be noticed more clearly by subjects who wondered why it was interrupted and generally reacted to it in a manner which made it perceptually more conspicuous and meaningful, resulting in the enhancement of its retention value.

More recently, in a comprehensive discussion of experiments in this area, Butterfield (1964) critically examined some of the methodological inadequacies involved in the use of interrupted task techniques for the study of selective recall. According to Butterfield, the inconsistent findings concerning selective recall of completed and incompleted tasks may stem from differential nature of tasks, instructions, personality, and developmental level of the subjects in the experiments.

C. *The Personality Type or Differential Position*

Some investigators have considered personality type an important variable in accounting for selective retention of pleasant and unpleasant experiences. In the absence of a general superiority of pleasant recall over unpleasant recall, it has been proposed that retention of pleasant or unpleasant experiences is determined by the personality type, or disposition, of the individual concerned. Taft (1954, p. 26) noted in this connection that:

> It is highly probable that differences in the findings of the various studies . . . are attributable to the type of subjects used. For example, some types of personality typically repress emotionally distressing experiences while others typically recall them.

One of the early advocates of this standpoint was Kowalewski (Rapaport, 1959, p. 43) who coined the concepts *memory optimism* and *memory pessimism* to explain the results of his questionnaire study. The group which remembered P events better than U events was considered by him as typical of the first memory type, whereas the group favoring U events was identified with the other memory type. According to Kowalewski, the majority of people are memory optimists. Subsequently, other investigators (e.g., Meltzer, 1930; O'Kelley and Steckle, 1940; Washburn *et al* 1925a, b; etc.) attempted to explain the phenomenon of selective recall in terms of concepts of different memory types suggested by Kowalewski. The obvious limitation of such concepts as memory optimism and memory pessimism, however, is that they are *ex-post-facto*, and, consequently, hopelessly circular. These two supposedly opposite personality types have neither been defined in operational terms nor measured or assessed on any objective basis by any of the above-mentioned investigators.

There have, however, been a number of studies (Abel, 1938; Belmont and Birch, 1951; Cartwright, 1942; Rosenthal, 1944; and Pachauri, 1936, for example) which have reported relationships between measured personality characteristic and selective patterns of recall. Atkinson (1953) suggested a resolution of the apparent contradiction between the Zeigarnik effect and the findings of many investigators (e.g., Glixman, 1949; Rosenzweig, 1943), who reported greater recall of completed than incompleted tasks, in terms of the "need achievement" (nAch) variable. He proposed that under conditions where achievement motivation was aroused, subjects low in nAch would recall more completed than incompleted tasks, whereas subjects high in nAch tended to recall more incompleted than completed tasks. Atkinson analyzed the personality dispositions of subjects used by Zeigarnik and by Marrow (1938a, b,) and concluded that these subjects were relatively high in need for achievement. Green (1963) demonstrated that a greater Zeigarnik effect was exhibited by volunteers than by nonvolunteers. Insofar as volunteers were suggested by Atkinson (1953) to be high in nAch, Green's results were consistent with Atkinson's contention. In another study, Atkinson and Raphelson (1956) replicated the finding that subjects high in nAch recalled more incompleted tasks than low nAch subjects under ego-orientation. However, under task orientation the two groups did not differ in their recall of incompleted tasks. Atkinson and Raphelson also observed that under task orientation, subjects high in need for affiliation (nAff) recalled more incompleted tasks than did low nAff subjects. Under ego-orientation the two affiliation groups did not differ significantly in their recall of incompleted tasks. These findings were explained in terms of subjects' motive structures as proposed by McClelland (1951). It has been assumed that high nAch subjects are success seekers and are motivated primarily by a need to approach success. On the other hand, low nAch subjects are failure avoiders and are motivated primarily by a need to avoid failure. Furthermore, ego-orienting instructions are assumed to enhance the motive state of the subjects. Such instructions therefore would increase avoidance-of-failure type behavior in low nAch subjects causing them to recall less incompleted tasks. Same instructions, however, would be seen as an incentive or challenge by high nAch subjects, and consequently would increase their approach to or recall of incompleted tasks. The achievement-motive theory has not been extended beyond establishing the relationship between incompleted tasks recall and nAch. For instance, the theory makes no prediction about the recall of completed tasks or of pleasant and unpleasant experiences that does not involve interruption paradigm.

Alper (1946a, b, 1948, 1952, 1957) and Eriksen (1954) have proposed alternative theoretical principles to accommodate diverse, and often contradictory, findings in this area. Both of them proposed that individual differences in ego-strength interacted with the experimental context of task-orientation versus ego-orientation to give rise to differential patterns of recall of affective items.

Alper (1948) questioned the general validity of Rosenzweig's (1943) functionalistic formulation that an ego-defensive situation would necessarily lead to greater P than U recall, and under a need-persistive state the pattern would be reversed in favor of U recall. Instead, Alper asserted that the patterns of selective recall would be influenced by personality variables such as ego-strength, self-esteem, and pride of the subjects. She recognized the differential effects of task-tension and ego-tension (or need-persistence and ego-defense as proposed by Rosenzweig) on selective recall but, without studying the role of this variable in isolation, Alper also considered the variable of personality type and attempted to determine the interaction between the two variables. In her theoretical formulations, all the possible patterns of interactions between two motivational contexts produced through task and ego-orienting instructions and different personality types as defined by herself in terms of ego-strength, have been accommodated. From the results of her study, Alper (1948) concluded that there were two major patterns of selective recall, and suggested the possibility of two additional patterns. The first pattern, she labeled as the "strong ego" pattern. This included those subjects who recalled more incompleted than completed tasks under task-orientation and recalled more completed than incompleted tasks under ego-orientation. It was assumed that task-orientation does not threaten and ego-orientation threatens the self-esteem of strong ego-individuals. Ambition and pride were suggested as the major personality characteristics of persons belonging to this category. As noted by Alper, this pattern of selective recall would be consistent with the findings of both Zeigarnik (1938) and Rosenzweig (1943). The second major pattern of selective recall suggested by Alper was the "weak-ego" pattern. This pattern was the reverse of the strong-ego pattern. The weak-ego individuals were characterized by low self-confidence, low self-esteem, and low frustration tolerance. Under task orientation, these individuals tended to boost their self-esteem and confidence by recalling more successfully completed tasks. This helped them to counteract their sense of failure. Under ego-orientation, however, they feel too threatened to counteract their failures and hence were forced to recognize their failure experiences. This tendency manifested itself in greater recall for incompleted tasks. According to Alper (pp. 132-3):

> The recall of incompleted tasks under conditions of competitive failure by individuals with weak self-esteem organization is dynamically very different, then, from the recall of incompleted tasks by strong egos under objectively non-stressful conditions. The recall of the latter group is consistent with Zeigarnik's task tension and Rosenzweig's need-persistive theory, while the recall of the former suggests a mechanism of defense which is more accurately described as ego-offense rather than ego defense. It is only under conditions where the threat to self-esteem is seen as potential but not as actual that weak egos can protect their tenuous self-esteem by recalling successfully completed tasks.

The third pattern suggested by Alper consisted of greater recall of completed tasks under both task- and ego-orientation. Individuals showing this recall pattern were characterized as insecure and narcissistic, and were in constant need to support their self-esteem. The fourth pattern of selective recall consisting of superior recall of incompleted tasks under both task- and ego-orientation was suggested as a logical possibility rather than as a demonstrated fact. Individuals belonging to this category would perhaps possess a very high degree of ego-strength and self-esteem, and would, therefore, experience their failures as challenges rather than ego-threats. Alper's theoretical formulation attempts to integrate the functionalistic approach of Rosenzweig and the personality-type position within a comprehensive conceptual framework.

Erikson's (1954) study provides further support to the idea that patterns of selective recall are determined by the interaction of experimental context or the subject's orientation and personality variables. Erikson found that under ego-orientation, individuals having high scores on the MMPI psychasthenia scale recalled more incompleted tasks than individuals having low scores on that scale and individuals having high scores on the MMPI hysteria scale recalled fewer incompleted tasks than the low scoring individuals on the scale. He also found that high ego-strength individuals recalled more incompleted tasks than low ego-strength individuals under ego-orientation. With respect to the recall of completed tasks, Erikson found no personality-related differences. Erikson's findings, however, were contradicted by Jourard (1954), who found no consistent relationship between ego-strength measure and selective recall of completed and incompleted tasks.

There have been other investigators who tried to determine the influence of another personality dimension, namely, introversion-extroversion, on selective recall. Studies that generally addressed themselves to the question of how introversion and extroversion might be related to the phenomenon of selective recall of interrupted and completed tasks or pleasant and unpleasant materials (e.g., Brown, 1961; Dodwell, 1964; Inglis, 1960; Kanungo, 1968) have failed to offer any conclusive answer. Kanungo (1968) tested the possibility that Eysenck's (1947) introversion-extroversion dimension may be independently related to selective recall of incompleted and completed tasks. According to Eysenck, extroverts are less socialized than normals and introverts are supposedly oversocialized. Undersocialization might lead extroverts to overestimate their successful performance in order to preserve or enhance their favorable self-image and to ignore failures in order to defend their self-esteem. Introverts, on the other hand, may tend to underestimate their successful performance and be preoccupied by failures. On this basis, Eriksen (1954, p. 49) hypothesized that extroverts "would be expected to recall relatively more completed than incompleted tasks while for the introversive subjects this tendency would be reversed". Kanungo's (1968) results failed to support Eriksen's predictions. His results showed that both introverts and extroverts recalled greater number of incompleted (failure) than completed experiences under task-orientation. Under ego-orientation, no difference between successfully completed and incompleted experience was observed in each of the two groups. In a discussion of "mediation-avoidance hypothesis" (Inglis, 1960), Butterfield (1964, p. 317) derived the following predictions regarding the recall of unsuccessful or incompleted (I) task only:

1. Under conditions of low stress, introverts recall fewer I tasks than extroverts.
2. Under conditions of high stress, introverts recall more I tasks than extroverts.
3. If both the introverts and extroverts are neurotic the differences predicted in Hypothesis 1 and 2 above are greater than if the groups are unselected for neuroticism.
4. Under similar instructional conditions, there are no mean differences between neurotic and stable groups which are equal on or unselected for introversion-extroversion.
5. Under similar instructional conditions, the variance is greater and the distribution of avoidance scores is more bimodal for neurotic than for stable groups when the groups are equal on extroversion-introversion.

If it is assumed that high nAch is an index of neurotic extroversion, hypotheses 1 and 2 find indirect support from the findings of Atkinson (1953), Atkinson and Raphelson (1956), and Caron and Wallach (1959). However, the results of Kanungo (1968) that tested directly the hypotheses, failed to support them. Hypothesis 3 has not been tested even indirectly and, as Butterfield points out, hypotheses 4 and 5 have not received any empirical support.

Overall, the studies on the role of personality variables such as nAch, ego-strength, or extroversion-introversion in selective recall concern themselves with selective recall of only incompleted or unpleasant experiences in which ego-threatening or anxiety-producing mediators are in operation. They prove to be inadequate in explaining selective recall of completed or pleasant experiences. Furthermore, as Butterfield (1964) points out, the relationship among various personality constructs such as nAch and ego-strength, or ego-strength and extroversion remains in question. As a final comment, it may be stated that the diverse research literature representing a differential personality-type position does not yet permit any definitive statement regarding selective recall of both P and U affective experiences as a function of personality dispositions. It is generally recognized that personality dispositions are very likely to influence the way individuals respond to affective experiences, thereby affecting their selective recall; however, the exact nature and extent of such influences under diverse conditions are yet to be determined conceptually and empirically.

D. *The Contextual Position*

Barrett (1938) was one of the first investigators in this area who noted the influence of emotional set on retention of affective materials. In her experiment mentioned earlier she observed that a group of subjects anticipating an examination remembered U materials better than P materials. She conducted experiments to study the effects of such "mental sets" in more detail and concluded that superiority of P recall found in most of the experiments, including her own, might be explained in terms of a "happy frame of mind" on the part of the subjects. The view expressed by McGeoch and Irion (1952) is quite consistent with this proposition. According to them, "a current irritability may condition selection and emphasis of U items and a current expectancy of good fortune may condition an emphasis on P items" (p. 387).

Edwards (1942) developed the concept of "frame of reference" and specified its influence on selective retention from a comprehensive theoretical viewpoint. Seeking to resolve the differences in interpretation of the role of affectivity in remembering and forgetting, Edwards restated the problem of differential forgetting of affective materials in terms of the "frame of reference" of an individual. According to Edwards, neither the quality nor the magnitude of affect was the crucial variable influencing retention in these studies. Differential retention of affective materials would have to be explained in terms of whether the materials learned conformed to an individual's existing frame of reference, i.e., his motivational system including his attitudes and values. Edwards, therefore, suggested that if we could determine an individual's frame of reference, we would be able to predict which experiences would tend to be remembered. Edwards's own study (1941) on memory for political views lent support to his hypothesis. The studies by Alper and Korchin (1952), Jones and Aneshansel (1956), Kanungo and Das (1960), Levine and Murphy (1943), and Taft (1954), also appeared to support Edwards's viewpoint.

Osgood (1953, pp. 571 ff.), in an attempt to resolve the conflicting evidences for and against Freudian repression hypothesis, proposed a distinction between two kinds of affective materials—those having *judged* affect and those having *felt* affect. According to Osgood, the repression hypothesis can explain selective recall of only those experiences that have felt affect for the individual and not of those experiences that have only judged affect. Edwards's frame of reference hypothesis has been considered better in explaining selective recall of experiences having judged but not felt affect (Kanungo and Das, 1960). However, the question has been raised as to whether the two hypotheses are necessary to account for selective retention of affective materials—one for felt affect and the other for judged affect. Kanungo and Dutta (1966) have tried to answer this question. According to them, Osgood's distinction between the two types of affect assumes that an individual may judge certain stimuli as pleasant or unpleasant, but may not feel about the stimuli in the same way. A closer scrutiny would reveal that both intellectual judgment and feeling are two aspects of the same perceptual process involved in an individual's experience. The individual experiences stimuli with different degrees of emotional involvement and not, as Osgood thinks, sometimes at the intellectual level and sometimes at the emotional level. When a subject is asked to rate an adjective itself as "pleasant" or "unpleasant", his emotional involvement is minimal, offering greater scope for rational judgment. Compared to this situation, his emotional involvement would increase and the scope for rational judgment would decrease when he is rating some intimate personal experience. In fact, every experience, even the one Osgood considers as having felt affect, is also judged by the individual to be either pleasant or unpleasant. Such judgments, however, are more influenced by personal sentiment than rational considerations. In each case, the individual's judgments about stimuli have to be relied upon because those are the only available indicators of his experiences. The following example will make the point clear. Osgood would claim that a stimulus word such as *swindler,* when perceived as an attribute of an opponent is naturally expected to be judged by an individual as extremely unpleasant. At the same time, however, the individual may feel a pleasant experience since the word characterizes his opponent. This was, however, interpreted differently by Kanungo and Dutta, who argued that these two experiences refer to two totally different situations. Perceiving the stimulus word attributed to the opponent as unpleasant and perceiving one's experience of such a situation as pleasant, are two independent experiences. Hence, the individual here is not perceiving one and the same thing. Judging one's feeling about the external stimulus word in a certain context is one thing and judging one's feeling about the inner experience with regard to the whole situation is another. In the former case he is perceiving the affective tone of the stimulus word itself when presented in a certain context. In the latter case he is reflecting on the affective tone of his own experience of the total situation. Here again in each case the individual is judging the affective tone. Thus the duality between experiences having judged and felt affect is more apparent than real. Hence for the sake of parsimony, the two explanations offered for their retention need reformulation.

Kanungo and Dutta (1966) critically examined Edwards's hypothesis and contested any essential distinction claimed by Edwards between the hedonistic hypothesis of Freud and his own frame of reference hypothesis. They contended that individual frame of reference was a motivational concept, and that it was therefore legitimate to assume a necessary and direct relationship between compatibility with one's frame of reference and pleasant emotion as well as between incompatibility with this frame and unpleasant emotion. Thus, compatibility-incompatibility and pleasantness-unpleasantness were suggested as highly overlapping, if not identical, dimensions. Edwards intended to refute the hedonistic contention, particularly of the Freudian variety, by affirming that pleasant experiences incompatible with one's frame of reference would be remembered less well than the compatible experiences. For instance, Edwards suggested that although fulfillment of a sexual desire is a pleasant experience, one may refrain from indulging in prohibited sexual acts (or may forget such experiences) in order to conform to the social values contained in their frame of reference. Likewise, an unpleasant experience (unfulfilled sexual desire in this case) may be quite compatible with one's frame of reference (conforming to one's social conscience, in this case), and may be easily recalled. What Edwards described as compatibility and incompatibility of an experience with one's frame of reference was only "a matter of determining the presence or absence of conflict of this particular experience in terms of individual's values" (p. 50). But congruence of an experience, as a whole, with the set of values, attitudes, and desires is necessarily compatible with this frame of reference and will evoke, on the whole, a pleasant affect. On the other hand, an experience that is in conflict with this motivational frame will result in unpleasant affect. For example, in the Kanungo and Das (1960) study, when a favorable stereotype was attributed to one's own group, it was obviously perceived as compatible with one's motivational frame. Due to this compatibility, the total situation was experienced by him as pleasant. On the other hand, an unfavorable stereotype when attributed to one's own group was perceived as incompatible with this frame and led him to perceive the total situation as unpleasant. When the stereotypes were ascribed to the rival group, the affective pattern was just the reverse. This suggests that compatibility-incompatibility and pleasantness-unpleasantness can be considered as highly overlapping phenomena, and, therefore, Edwards's hypothesis can hardly be considered as other than a restatement of the hedonistic position, i.e., P material will be recalled better than U material. Thus Edwards's explanation appears to be no more adequate than the hedonistic position, whether of Freudian variety or otherwise, as an account for experimental data in this area. McGeoch and Irion (1952) have noted in this connection that ". . . of course, on the whole, experiences which agree with one's frame of reference are judged to be P and those which do not are judged to be U" (p. 387).

A more recent version of the "contextual" or the "frame of reference" approach has been proposed by Feather (1969). According to him, under standard free recall conditions individuals will report more experiences that are consistent with their attitudes than experiences that are inconsistent with their attitudes. His results supported the theoretical assumption that balanced attitude structures "will be more likely to survive in memory than unbalanced attitude structures" (p. 317). Feather's position is very similar to that of Edwards except that he uses balance theory (Heider, 1958) for explaining the selective recall phenomena. Edwards's concept of compatibility-incompatibility and Feather's balanced-imbalanced structure refer to one and the same dimension. Like a compatible experience, an experience keyed to a balanced attitudinal structure will be experienced as pleasant in affect. Conversely, an experience that produces imbalance (or incompatibility) will be experienced as unpleasant in affect. Thus by saying that balanced attitude structures are retained better than unbalanced ones, Feather has only restated the Freudian position that pleasant experiences are retained better than unpleasant.

E. *Retroactive Inhibition Position*

Another explanation for superiority of P over U recall was suggested by Stagner (1931) who interpreted rapid forgetting of U materials as compared to P materials in terms of retroactive inhibition. Stagner assumed that unpleasantness involved some kind of incomplete situation which evoked different inappropriate and competing responses; interference due to the presence of such competing responses would thus lower the recall value of any previously experienced unpleasant material.

The implications of Stagner's position, which asserts that all unpleasant experiences involve a perceived state of incompletion are thus susceptible to retroactive interference, have yet to be investigated in theoretical terms. It is to be noted, however, that Stagner's explanation is quite contradictory to the findings and explanations of Zeigarnik (1938). According to the latter investigator, incompletion creates a state of quasi-need within the individual, and persistence of such a need or·state of tension accounts for greater recall of uncompleted tasks than of completed ones. The concept of retroactive inhibition suggested by Stagner, on the other hand, argues in favor of greater recall of completed than of uncompleted tasks. In view of their conflicting viewpoints, explanations offered by Stagner and Zeigarnik are difficult to reconcile.

Recently, several investigators (D'Zurilla, 1965; Holmes, 1972; Holmes and Schallow, 1969) who have suggested that response interference or competition may account for the reduced recall of unpleasant experiences following ego-threat. D'Zurilla, for instance, found that subjects under ego-threat condition entertained more additional thoughts that were irrelevant to the recall task, than did control subjects. These irrelevant thoughts may have acted as interfering cognitive events to reduce the recall of U materials. In a more direct test of interference theory, Holmes (1972) found that any information concerning subject's personality (regardless of whether the information was ego-enhancing or ego-threatening) may interfere with recall of other unrelated experiences. According to Holmes, selective recall of either pleasant or unpleasant experiences can be explained in terms of poor retrieval due to subject's attention to his own emotional states that act as interfering cognitive events. It may be noted that within the purview of interference explanation of selective recall, two different mechanisms have been suggested. Holmes (1972), for instance, has argued in favor of attention-interference mechanism, and D'Zurilla (1965), like Stagner, has talked of response competition mechanism. While both the mechanisms may influence selective recall of affective materials, the conditions under which one or the other mechanism becomes operative is an issue that needs to be settled before interference theory can be considered viable.

The five theoretical positions discussed in this chapter assumed that variation in affective quality of experiences is responsible, at least in part, for their selective retention, although each of them proposed a different mechanism to explain the observed relationship between the affective quality of experiences and their retention. However, several investigators have questioned the validity of any position which asserts a differential retention of pleasant and unpleasant experiences on the basis of their affective quality. Instead, they have proposed the hypothesis that affective intensity of experiences, regardless of their quality, can be considered as the major determinant of their selective retention. In the following chapter, a comprehensive account of the intensity hypothesis, its main characteristics, and a comparative discussion of the earlier as opposed to the current version of the hypothesis, will be presented.

CHAPTER 3

The Intensity Hypothesis

Several researchers consider intensity rather than quality of experiences as the major determinant of their retention. One of the early advocates of such a standpoint was Lipmann (1911), cited in Rapaport (1959, pp. 54-58), who held that the vividness of memory varied with the intensity of memory traces and that forgetting was a matter of disappearance of these traces. In his survey of free association experiments in the area of crime detection, Lipmann emphasized the significant role of what he called an "interest tone" of an experience in determining the intensity of memory traces. Lipmann used the concept of "interest tone" in the same sense as "emotional tone." He suggested that emotionally loaded perception complexes create especially intense memory traces that are less likely to disappear rapidly and are more likely to be revived easily. Rapaport (1959, p. 65) also reported a study of Wuerdemann which concluded that experiences with weak and superficial feeling tone would be forgotten more easily than those of great feeling, intensity, and depth.

Jersild (1931) suggested that better recall for P than U experiences as observed by many investigators including himself might depend ultimately on the affective intensity of the memories. He proposed that in order to be relieved of an unpleasant feeling an individual would tend to reduce its intensity and this would lead to less stable traces for unpleasant memory experiences as compared to the pleasant ones. Jersild's notion of a subjective reduction of initially perceived intensity of affect by some remedial mechanism could be considered as consistent with the concept of "reduction of cognitive dissonance" formulated by Festinger (1963) as well as with the "shift toward congruence" proposed and developed by Osgood (Osgood *et al.*, 1957; Osgood and Tannenbaum, 1955). The similarity of Peters's (Rapaport, 1959, p. 52) proposition regarding "diminishing displeasure in consciousness" to these viewpoints should also be noted in this connection.

The notion of a subjective reduction of perceived intensity of affect of unpleasant experiences has also been supported in a recent study by Holmes

(1970). Holmes not only found that "experiences which decreased in affective intensity between the time they occurred and the time at which they were to be recalled were less likely to be recalled than those that did not decrease in intensity"; he also found that "over time unpleasant experiences decreased more in intensity of their affect than pleasant experiences" (p. 234). Holmes suggested several processes that may be responsible for the reduction of affect of unpleasant experiences. For example, as Stagner (1931) has observed, most unpleasant experiences may represent things about which something has to be done. And it is quite possible that, generally, during the retention interval something is done in order to alleviate the tension or reduce the intensity of affect associated with the experience. This explanation, however, is very similar to the "dissonance reduction" concept proposed by Festinger and his associates. Another interesting explanation suggested by Holmes to explain the phenomenon is in terms of attitudinal effect of *mere exposure* (Zajonc, 1968). Zajonc has demonstrated that "mere repeated exposure of an individual to a stimulus object enhances his attitude toward it" in the favorable direction. Several studies (Menzies, 1935; Waters and Leeper, 1936) suggest that affectively more pleasant and unpleasant experiences are thought of more frequently during retention interval than are affectively more neutral experiences. If this is the case, then over time the unpleasant experiences would tend to become more and more neutral and pleasant experiences would tend to become more and more pleasant. However, till the present time, none of the above explanations has been adequately tested.

Among the many experiments on the recall of P, U, and N experiences, there are some which reported that P and U experiences were equally recalled and that both were better remembered than N experiences (Barlow, 1955; Cason, 1932; Chaney and Lauer, 1929; Klugman, 1956; Menzies, 1933, 1935; Turner and Barlow, 1951; Waters and Leeper, 1936; White and Ratliff, 1934). In general, authors of these experiments have postulated that the determinant of retention is the intensity of affect rather than its quality. In Weiner's (1966b, p. 28) words:

> There does seem to be evidence that the intensity of affect at the time an event occurs is related to subsequent recall. The data concerning the association between the quality of affect and memory is less substantial.

On the basis of an extensive review of studies in this area, Rapaport (1959) also tends to favor affective intensity rather than affective quality as the determinant of selective retention.

The Main Characteristics of the Hypothesis

At this point it is difficult to see how the various quality of affect hypotheses or theoretical positions as described in the earlier chapter and the intensity of affect hypothesis as described in this chapter can be integrated into a generalized framework. In various theoretical positions the empirical findings supporting them often appear contradictory and at times mutually exclusive. For instance, it seems quite evident that neither Rozenzweig's (1943) findings can be explained by simple frame of reference or contextual approach of Edwards (1942), nor the differential or "personality type" position can explain the findings reported as supporting contextual position (Kanungo and Das, 1960, for example). This creates a need for working toward a more comprehensive approach to selective memory phenomena. In this context, the theoretical implications of the intensity hypothesis are quite far-reaching. Although several studies have suggested intensity of affect as an explanatory mechanism, no systematic attempt has been made as yet to relate it to other contextual and personality variables and thus to integrate it with other theoretical positions. Such an attempt is made in this book.

Apart from inquiries into the effects of a number of variables such as personal relevance, context, personality type, etc., on selective memory for affective materials, the book will report in some detail several investigations of the role of *perceived intensity of affect per se* in selective memory. It may be pointed out that a conceptual distinction can be made between *perceived* intensity of affect and *normative* intensity of affect of stimulus materials that are committed to memory. The former is determined by the response made by a single individual who is tested for his memory, whereas the latter is determined through the use of a standardization procedure using groups different from those tested for memory.

Several laboratory studies have tested memory for materials varying in normative affect and have shown that both the normative quality (Amster, 1964) and the normative intensity (Windgard, 1966) can affect memory process. The investigations reported in this book, however, do not deal with normative affect. They limit themselves to the effects of only perceived intensity of affect. Thus the book reaffirms the modified version of intensity hypothesis and asks the question whether other factors remaining constant, the intensity of perceived affect rather than its quality, acts as the immediate antecedent determinant of selective learning and retention. The perceived affective intensity may be considered as an intervening organismic variable which, on the one hand, is dependent upon the antecedent variables such as motivational involvement, attitudes, personality characteristics of the individual, and, on the other hand, is directly influencing the nature of his learning and retention processes. In other words, it may reasonably be hypothesized that an individual perceives an affective material, whether pleasant or unpleasant, as more or less intense than some other materials due to the influence of any of the following major factors, either in isolation or in combination:

(1) The context in which he finds himself.
(2) The level of his motivational involvement.
(3) The organismic predispositions such as attitudinal and personality variables.

Thus there might be a number of such factors due to which an affective experience is perceived by the individual as more or less intense than some others. But, theoretically, it would be important not only to demonstrate this, but also to seek an answer to the simple question whether the greater perceived intensity of affect of an experience, for whatever reasons, would make it more "retainable" for the individual.

Several studies (Rozenzweig, 1943) reviewed in the preceding chapter reveal that in task-oriented context unpleasant materials tends to be recalled better than pleasant materials, and in ego-oriented context this direction gets reversed. But it can be argued, as has been done in the subsequent chapters of this book, that under these experimental contexts the respective perceived intensities of pleasant and unpleasant materials get changed, and these changes in perceived intensity of affect of materials that act as intervening variable can explain the nature of context effects on selective recall. Likewise, extending the perceived intensity hypothesis to personality-type theoretical framework (Alper, 1952), it may be argued that the different patterns of interaction between the variables of context and "personality types" not only lead to differential recall of pleasant and unpleasant materials, but also may lead to differential patterns of perceived affective intensity of pleasant and unpleasant materials. Here again the perceived intensity of affect as experienced by the individual for whatever internal or environmental reasons, may be the immediate antecedent determinant of selective retention. Furthermore, the concept "selective retention or memory" includes two separate processes—selective learning and selective retrieval. The study of the effects of perceived intensity of affect on both selective learning and retrieval mechanism will be of considerable theoretical interest.

To sum up, the perceived intensity of affect hypothesis can be formulated in the following way: other factors remaining constant, intensity of feeling tone of an experience, irrespective of its quality, as perceived by the individual under different degrees of emotional involvement in whatever context, is the immediate antecedent determinant of both selective learning and retrieval processes. The implications of this general hypothesis for selective learning have been explored in four different experiments reported in Chapter 4. In Chapter 5 the implications of intensity hypothesis for selective retrieval mechanism have been dealt with at some length in the discussion of three other experiments.

CHAPTER 4

Intensity of Perceived Affect and Selective Learning and Retention

Intensity of Perceived Affect and Frame of Reference Explanation

The contextual or frame of reference explanation of selective memory as advanced by Edwards (1942) was discussed in Chapter 2. It was suggested that although several studies (Edwards, 1941: Kanungo and Das, 1960; Levine and Murphy, 1943) claim to provide empirical support for Edwards's formulation as opposed to alternative Freudian principle of repression (Freud, 1925), the two formulations—frame of reference and repression—at least as explanatory devices of selective memory, are not that much different from one another. In his frame of reference explanation, Edwards has only restated the same proposition implied in Freudian concept of repression that pleasant experiences are learned and retained better than unpleasant experiences. Furthermore, Osgood's (1953) distinction between materials having judged affect and materials having felt affect was shown to be more apparent than real, and hence his argument in favor of invoking frame of reference explanations for studies dealing with felt affect seemed no more durable.

In view of this, it was thought more parsimonious and desirable to invoke intensity of perceived affect hypothesis as a single explanatory principle to deal with the results of studies that use frame of reference paradigm. Thus it was argued that an individual may enter different contexts that determine his frame of reference under different degrees of emotional involvement or arousal. The degree of the perceived affective tones of materials experienced in these contexts may systematically undergo changes as a joint function of different degrees of emotional involvement and particular frame of reference evoked in him. The changes in the perceived intensity of affect then in turn may determine selective learning and retention of the materials.

Two separate experiments were conducted to test these possibilities.

Experiment I†

An experimental paradigm similar to an earlier study (Kanungo and Das, 1960) was used to produce two levels of emotional involvement. Subjects were selected from a linguistic group in India (Bengali) known to have strong feeling of group identification and pride. Four sets of adjectives were used as materials to be retained. Subjects were randomly assigned to four different groups in each of which they had to undergo four different stages schematically presented in Table 1. Subjects first rated the affectivity of two sets of adjectives during the initial rating stage. In the second stage of report reading, subjects learned two other sets of adjectives—one as attributes of their own group (Bengali) and the other as attributes of a fictitious group (Lampani). During the third stage of final rating, subjects rated the affective tone of adjectives they learned during the second stage. It was thought that the subjects would perceive the adjectives under greater emotional involvement when these were ascribed to Bengalis than when these were ascribed to Lampanis. In the fourth stage of free recall, subjects' recall for adjectives learned and rated during the second and third stages, respectively, were tested.

Table 1. *Schematic Presentation of Four Stages of the Experiment*

	Initial rating	Report reading		Final rating		Free recall	
		Bengali	Lampani	Bengali	Lampani	Bengali	Lampani
Report 1 (R_1)[a]	Sets III and IV	Set I (R_1)	Set II	Set I	Set II	Set I	Set II
Report 2 (R_2)	Sets I and II	Set III (R_2)	Set IV	Set III	Set IV	Set III	Set IV
Report 3 (R_3)	Sets III and IV	Set II (R_3)	Set I	Set II	Set I	Set II	Set I
Report 4 (R_4)	Sets I and II	Set IV (R_4)	Set III	Set IV	Set III	Set IV	Set III

[a] $n = 20$ in each group.

Hypothesis

It was proposed that the degree of the affective tone of materials changes when experienced in different degrees of emotional involvement and that such intensity of affect as perceived by the individual determines retention. Three hypotheses relating changes in perceived intensity of affect of adjectives were derived after congruity principles (Osgood and Tannenbaum,

†Experiments I and II were previously reported by Kanungo and Dutta (1966). Copyright (1966) by the American Psychological Association. Portions of the previous report are reprinted by permission.

1955), and two more hypotheses were formulated with respect to selective recall of such adjectives. The hypotheses are as follows:

1. The intensity of affect of pleasant adjectives will be greater than those of the unpleasant adjectives when ascribed to one's own group.
2. There will be no difference between the respective intensities of affect of pleasant and unpleasant adjectives when ascribed to a fictitious group.
3. The intensity of affect of a pleasant adjective when ascribed to one's own group will be greater as compared to the intensity of affect of the same adjective ascribed to a fictitious group; the intensity of affect of an unpleasant adjective when ascribed to one's own group will be less as compared to the intensity of the same adjective when ascribed to the fictitious group.
4. Recall will be directly determined by the intensity of affect as perceived by the subjects; thus more pleasant adjectives than unpleasant ones will be recalled when ascribed to one's own group. No difference between the recalls of pleasant and unpleasant adjectives are expected when these are ascribed to a fictitious group.
5. Mean intensity of affect of the adjectives recalled will be higher than mean intensity of affect of the items not recalled. This will hold true for both pleasant and unpleasant adjectives and irrespective of the contexts in which they are presented.

Method

Subjects and materials. Eighty Bengali undergraduate students volunteered to serve as subjects. One hundred adjectives in the Bengali language were given to 40 judges to rate each of them for its frequency of usage and degree of pleasantness or unpleasantness. The frequency of usage was measured in terms of a unipolar five-point scale with verbally labeled categories. Degree of affect, on the other hand, was measured on a bipolar five-point scale ranging from extremely pleasant to extremely unpleasant. Intensity of affect for any particular adjective was determined by taking its mean polarity score. Four sets (I, II, III, IV) of 10 adjectives were chosen from the sample of 100. Each set consisted of five pleasant and five unpleasant adjectives. Within each set the pleasant and unpleasant adjectives were matched as far as possible for frequency and intensity of affect. The English equivalents of these sets are presented in Table 2.

Separate booklets were prepared, one containing adjectives from sets I and II and the other containing those from sets III and IV. Every adjective in a booklet appeared four times to be rated on four bipolar-nine-point scales, such as, unpleasant-pleasant, good-bad, attractive-repulsive, and unacceptable-acceptable. The bipolar scales were printed below the adjectives with verbally labeled categories such as extreme, strong, moderate, mild, neutral. Four different randomly determined sequences of presentation of these 20 adjectives were used for four different scales. Care was taken to present in varied sequence the four different scales to different subjects.

Table 2. *Sets of Pleasant and Unpleasant Adjectives with their Rated Frequency of Usage and Intensity of Affect*

Set	P adjectives	Mean frequency of use	Mean intensity of affect	U adjectives	Mean frequency of use	Mean intensity of affect
I	Polite	4.64	1.12	Effeminate	4.20	0.88
	Idealist	3.84	1.36	Lazy	4.40	1.16
	Modest	4.36	1.24	Sectarian	4.16	1.52
	Intelligent	4.96	1.60	Nervous	4.68	1.32
	Judicious	4.28	1.28	Dirty	4.80	1.88
II	Sincere	4.40	1.36	Rude	3.72	1.40
	Witty	4.68	1.32	Cruel	3.88	1.56
	Honest	4.72	1.88	Orthodox	4.44	1.16
	Peace-loving	4.32	0.92	Miserly	4.56	1.80
	Self-confident	3.68	1.52	Crude	3.56	1.52
III	Kind	4.52	1.76	Stubborn	4.28	1.16
	Compassionate	4.16	1.52	Ungrateful	4.60	1.80
	Cooperative	3.76	0.92	Timid	4.36	1.32
	Refined	4.16	1.48	Shy	4.24	1.60
	Sociable	4.68	1.72	Intolerant	3.64	0.08
IV	Simple	4.64	0.88	Uncivil	4.92	1.76
	Self-dependent	4.20	1.60	Coarse	4.08	1.20
	Perseverent	3.80	1.28	Ignorant	4.08	1.38
	Brave	4.72	1.68	Autocratic	4.12	1.40
	Progressive	3.88	1.60	Disorderly	4.60	1.64

Four reports were prepared in the Bengali language (R_1, R_2, R_3, and R_4). Each of the reports contained at the top the following introduction:

> Given below are two translated extracts from the research reports published in the *International Bureau of Ethnic Research Bulletin* (Vol. 5, No. 17). The typical racial-cultural characteristics of two different socio-linguistic communities, namely, Bengali and Lampani (an Australian tribe) have been pointed out in the report. You might be interested in knowing them.

The rest of the contents of the four reports were different from each other with respect to adjectives attributed to Bengali and a fictitious Lampani group, respectively.

In R_1, set I adjectives were ascribed to Bengalis and set II adjectives were ascribed to Lampanis. R_2 contained set III adjectives ascribed to Bengalis and set IV adjectives ascribed to Lampanis. R_3 contained sets I and II, but these were ascribed to the two communities in a manner reverse to that of R_1. Likewise, R_4 contained sets III and IV, but these were ascribed to the two communities in a manner reverse to that of R_2.

Procedure. Subjects were randomly assigned to four groups of 20 subjects in each. During the initial rating stage, two of these groups ($n = 40$) were presented with booklets containing adjectives of sets I and II, and the remaining two groups ($n = 40$) were presented with booklets containing adjectives of sets III and IV. All of the subjects were instructed to rate each adjective in the respective booklets on the evaluative scale that appeared below the adjective by underlining the appropriate labeled category of the scale. Since each booklet contained four different evaluative scales on which each of the adjectives was to be rated, subjects rated each adjective four times.

After the subjects completed their ratings, the booklets were collected from them. One of the two groups who rated sets III and IV adjectives earlier was presented with R_1 and the other group was presented with R_3. Of the two remaining groups who rated sets I and II adjectives during the initial rating stage, one was presented with R_2 and the other was presented with R_4 (see Table 1). Subjects were asked to read the report.

After the report-reading stage had been completed, each subject was presented with a random listing of the adjectives which had been embedded in the material he had read previously. The subject was asked to rate these adjectives on each of the four evaluative scales in a similar manner to that of the initial rating. The booklets this time, however, not only contained an adjective with a scale below it as described earlier for the initial rating stage, but by the side of each adjective there also appeared the name of the community to specify to whom it was ascribed in the report. Thus for each subject, each adjective that appeared in the report earlier also appeared four times associated with either Bengali or Lampani as the case may be in a random sequence. Care was taken to avoid giving any impression to the subject that he would be asked to recall these adjectives later.

The booklets were collected after the subjects' ratings were over. Then the subject was given a recall sheet containing two columns—one for Bengali and the other for Lampani. He was allowed 5 minutes for free recall and was asked to write down as many adjectives as he could recall separately for Bengali and Lampani. The subject was free to recall either Bengali or Lampani adjectives as they occurred to him. The adjectives required of him to recall were those contained in the report and appeared in the booklet during his subsequent ratings. A 24-hour delayed recall was obtained from the subjects in the manner similar to that of immediate recall.

Results

In the initial rating stage of the experiment, 40 subjects rated the 10 P and 10 U adjectives of sets III and IV and another 40 subjects rated the 10 P and

Table 3. *Comparisons of Intensity of Affect of Pleasant and Unpleasant Adjectives During Initial and Final Rating*

	Initial	Final rating: Bengali	Final rating: Lampani	t
Experiment I				
P adjectives				
M	2.639	2.781	2.575	2.73**
SD	0.616	0.671	0.716	
U adjectives				
M	-2.631	-2.588	-2.806	3.01***
SD	0.592	0.744	0.575	
t	0.346	1.99*	3.15***	
		Kasanda	Lampani	
Experiment II				
P adjectives				
M	2.788	2.900	2.817	1.06
SD	0.917	0.962	0.961	
U adjectives				
M	-2.790	-2.906	-2.815	1.15
SD	1.128	0.985	0.966	
t	0.200	0.076	0.026	

* $p < 0.05$. ** $p < 0.02$. *** $p < 0.001$.

10 U adjectives of sets I and II. Thus, each of the 20 P and 20 U adjectives was rated by 40 subjects on four bipolar scales. The subjects' rating responses were transformed into ordinal weights. Neutral point on the scale was assigned a value of 0, and the mild, moderate, strong, and extreme points were assigned 1, 2, 3, and 4, respectively, with positive signs when the points appeared on the positive side of the pole and with negative signs when they appeared on the negative side of the pole. Mean intensity rating was calculated for each adjective based on the ratings of 40 subjects on four scales. Finally, the averages of such mean intensity ratings of 20 P and 20 U adjectives were calculated separately. Results presented in Table 3 reveal that during the initial rating stage the mean intensity ratings of P and U adjectives do not differ ($t = 0.346$).

During the final rating stage, each adjective from sets I, II, III, and IV when ascribed to Bengali was rated by subjects in R_1, R_3, R_2, and R_4 groups, respectively, and when ascribed to Lampani by subjects from R_3, R_1, R_4, and R_2 groups, respectively. Thus the mean intensity rating in the case of each adjective was calculated from the ratings of 20 subjects on four scales.

The averages of mean intensity ratings of 20 P and 20 U adjectives when ascribed to Bengali and Lampani are presented in Table 3. The results reveal that when ascribed to Bengali, the P adjectives are considered to have more intense affect that the U adjectives (t = 1.99, $p < 0.05$). When the adjectives are ascribed to Lampani, the opposite trend is noticed; the U adjectives are considered more intense in affect as compared to P adjectives (t = 3.15, $p <$ 0.001). These results support hypothesis 1 that when ascribed to one's own group, the intensities of affect of P adjectives will be greater than those of U adjectives. Hypothesis 2, however, is not supported. It was expected that no difference would be observed between the intensities of affect of P and U adjectives. Contrary to this expectation, the study revealed a significant difference between them. The mean intensity of affect of U adjectives was found to be greater than the mean intensity of affect of P adjectives when ascribed to Lampani.

Comparison of mean intensities of affect of P adjectives under the Bengali and Lampani conditions reveals that the former is significantly more intense than the latter (t = 2.73, $p < 0.02$). Similar comparison between the mean intensities of affect of U adjectives shows that when the adjectives are ascribed to Lampani the intensity of affect is significantly greater than when the adjectives are ascribed to Bengali (t = 3.01, $p < 0.01$). This supports hypothesis 3.

A two-way analysis of variance was used to analyze the recall scores of immediate as well as delayed recall tests. One of the two classifications was adjectives attributed to Bengali and to Lampani. The other classification was P and U adjectives. In immediate recall there seems to be no significant difference in the recall of P and U adjectives (F = 2.792, d.f. = 1/316, $p <$ 0.05). However, the F-ratios for the main effect of Bengali-Lampani and the interaction effect are significant beyond the 0.01 level (F = 12.849, d.f. = 1/316; and F = 24.216, d.f. = 1/316, respectively). Delayed recall was obtained from 73 subjects out of a total of 80 subjects who participated in immediate recall. In delayed recall, both the main effects and the interaction effect are significant at the 0.01 level (F = 6.662, d.f. = 1/288 in case of each of the main effects, and F = 8.824, d.f. = 1/288 in the case of the interaction effect).

The means of the number of adjectives recalled in each of the cells of 2 X 2 classification are presented in Table 4. It will be observed that both in immediate and delayed recall, subjects recalled more adjectives ascribed to Bengali than those ascribed to Lampani. This is quite consistent with the expectation that materials having greater relevance to the subjects would

Table 4. *Recall of Pleasant and Unpleasant Adjectives Under Different Conditions*

	Immediate recall (n = 80)		Delayed recall (n = 73)	
	Bengali	Lampani	Bengali	Lampani
P adjectives				
Total recalled	177	88	132	75
M	2.213	1.100	1.808	1.055
SD	1.179	0.903	1.278	0.977
U adjectives				
Total recalled	143	157	128	132
M	1.788	1.963	1.753	1.808
SD	1.330	1.197	1.168	1.300

Note. Each S was presented with five P and five U adjectives attributed to each of the two communities.

stimulate their attention and interest to a greater extent as compared to materials having low degree of relevance to them. In other words, a subject is naturally expected to be more interested in what is being said about himself than he is in what is said about other people. Further, the significant interaction effects in both the recall tests partially support hypothesis 4. The results are consistent with the prediction that more P than U adjectives would be recalled when ascribed to one's own group. When the adjectives were ascribed to Lampani, hypothesis 4 predicted no significant difference between the recall of P and U adjectives. The results, however, reveal that under this condition more U adjectives are recalled than P adjectives. Here it may be pointed out that the pattern of recalls of adjectives in Table 4 is consistent with the pattern of ratings of their intensity of affect in Table 3. On the one hand, U adjectives were perceived as being more intense in affect and also were recalled more frequently than P adjectives when ascribed to Lampani. On the other hand, P adjectives were considered more intense in affect and were also more easily recalled than U adjectives when ascribed to Bengali.

More substantive support for the intensity hypothesis can be found from the test of hypothesis 5. Comparisons of mean intensities of affect of recalled and nonrecalled adjectives under various conditions in immediate recall are presented in Table 5. Consideration of P and U adjectives irrespective of whether they are attributed to Bengali or Lampani reveals that in each case the mean intensity of affect of recalled items is significantly higher than the mean intensity of affect of nonrecalled items. Similar analyses done for

Table 5. *Comparisons of Intensity of Affect of Recalled and Nonrecalled Items in Immediate Recall*

	Pleasant (P) adjectives				Unpleasant (U) adjectives				Combined (P + U) adjectives			
	n	M	SD	*t*	*n*	M	SD	*t*	*n*	M	SD	*t*
Experiment I												
Bengali (B)												
Recalled	177	2.935	0.884	2.880*	143	−2.678	1.057	1.273	320	2.820	0.974	3.109*
Nonrecalled	223	2.668	0.950		257	−2.538	1.050		480	2.598	1.008	
Lampani (L)												
Recalled	88	2.639	1.009	0.713	157	−2.952	0.801	2.874*	245	2.839	0.896	3.106*
Nonrecalled	312	2.557	0.941		243	−2.710	0.867		555	2.624	0.912	
Combined (BL)												
Recalled	265	2.837	0.937	3.277*	300	−2.821	0.943	2.851*				
Nonrecalled	535	2.603	0.946		500	−2.622	0.967					
Experiment II												
Kasanda (K)												
Recalled	81	3.037	0.785	1.700	91	−2.961	0.960	0.754	172	2.997	0.882	1.660
Nonrecalled	219	2.850	1.013		209	−2.869	1.009		428	2.859	1.012	
Lampani (L)												
Recalled	71	2.915	1.073	0.915	83	−2.915	0.896	1.160	154	2.915	0.982	1.560
Nonrecalled	229	2.786	0.900		217	−2.777	0.988		446	2.782	0.943	
Combined (KL)												
Recalled	152	2.980	0.933	1.900	174	−2.939	0.931	1.380				
Nonrecalled	448	2.817	0.959		426	−2.822	1.000					

Note. In experiment I the *n* column gives the total number of recalled or nonrecalled items over 80 Ss; in experiment II the *n* column gives the total number of recalled oı nonrecalled items over 60 Ss. Mean of combines (P + U) was calculated from the S's polarity of ratings disregarding algebraic signs.

* $p < 0.05$.

adjectives ascribed to Bengali and to Lampani irrespective of their quality of affect show similar trends in each case (see Table 5). However, when separate analyses were done for P and U adjectives ascribed to Bengali, in the case of U adjectives the intensity of affect of recalled items was not found to be significantly different from the intensity of affect of nonrecalled items (t = 1.273, $p > 0.05$). Separate analyses for P and U adjectives ascribed to Lampani reveal that in the case of P adjectives, no significant difference was obtained between the intensities of affect of recalled and nonrecalled items (t = 0.713). The mean intensities of affect presented in Table 5 show that though the differences are nonsignificant, the means of recalled items are higher than the means of nonrecalled items. Taking all recall scores for 80 subjects, it was observed that a total of 565 recalls were obtained as against 1035 nonrecalled items. The mean intensity of affect of recalled items calculated from the polarity of ratings disregarding algebraic signs is 2.828 (SD = 0.942). This is higher than the mean intensity of affect of nonrecalled items (M = 2.612, SD = 0.957). The difference is significant at 0.001 level (t = 4.32). Thus hypothesis 5 is supported by these results.

Empirical support was obtained for the contention that under greater emotional involvements, retention is related to intensity of affect. However, the study failed to confirm the hypothesis that P and U adjectives will not differ in their rated intensity of affect and consequently in their recallability when they are attributed to the fictitious Lampani group. It was thought that when the adjectives were ascribed to Lampani, subjects would experience them under a neutral nonego-involved situation similar to the initial rating stage. The results reveal that adjectives when ascribed to Lampani were not perceived in the same way as in the initial stage. Unpleasant adjectives were rated as more intense in affect (see Table 3) and better recalled (see Table 4) than P adjectives when attributed to Lampani. This shows that the study failed to provide conditions of least emotional involvement for subjects. Such failure was presumably due to the presentation of both reports on Lampani and Bengali together in the same ego-involved context. It seems that subjects experienced adjectives attributed to Lampani also under greater emotional involvement and perceived them in a contrasting context to their own group. The fictitious Lampani group was perceived as a rival or inferior to their own group. Thus, in the case of Bengali, P adjectives were considered by subjects as extremely pleasant and U adjectives were only moderately unpleasant. In the case of Lampani, on the other hand, as a contrast effect, the subjects reacted as if the P adjectives were only moderately pleasant and the U adjectives were extremely unpleasant.

Experiment II

Experiment II was performed to test the validity of the above explanation and to examine the relation of retention of affective materials to the intensity of their affect under conditions of least emotional involvement.

Method

Subjects. Sixty volunteer subjects were drawn from an undergraduate college in India and were randomly assigned to four groups of 15 subjects each.

Materials and procedure. The materials used and the procedure followed in experiment II was exactly similar to those of experiment I except that instead of adjectives ascribed to Bengali they were ascribed to another fictitious tribe from Africa, "Kasanda". Briefly, during the initial rating stage two groups of subjects ($n = 30$) rated adjectives from sets III and IV and another two groups of subjects ($n = 30$) rated adjectives from sets I and II on four different scales. During the report-reading stage, one of the two groups who rated sets III and IV earlier read R_1 and the other group read R_3. Of the two remaining groups who rated sets I and II earlier, one group read R_2 and the other read R_4.

Each of these reports was similar to the corresponding report used in experiment I except that the word "Bengali" was substituted by "Kasanda, an African tribe". After reading the report, subjects in each group were asked to rate the adjectives describing Kasanda and Lampani on four evaluative scales. Soon after the final rating, subjects were allowed 5 minutes for free recall of adjectives which they read in the reports on Lampani and Kasanda. This time no delayed recall was taken, since in experiment I similar pattern of recall was observed in both delayed and immediate recall.

Results and Discussion

The results were analyzed in the same manner as in experiment I. The averages of mean intensity ratings of 20 P and 20 U adjectives calculated separately from the initial ratings of 30 subjects on four scales, and the averages of the mean intensity ratings of 20 P and 20 U adjectives when ascribed to Kasanda and Lampani are present in Table 3. It may be noted that during the final rating stage the mean intensity rating of each adjective was based on the rating of 15 subjects on four scales. Insignificant t-values presented in Table 3 reveal that P and U adjectives do not differ with respect to their intensities of affect either during initial rating or during final rating stages. Comparison of these results with those of experiment I indicates that a neutral nonego-involved situation was presented to the subjects during the final rating stage by substituting Kasanda for Bengali. Both Kasanda and Lampani were fictitious communities and were presented in a nonego-involved context. Hence, the perceived intensities of affect of P and U adjectives do not differ significantly when attributed to either of the two communities. Thus, hypothesis 2 finds support from these results.

Analysis of variance of recall scores revealed that neither the difference in the recall of P and U adjectives nor the difference in the recall of adjectives attributed to Kasanda and Lampani reached significance level ($F = 1.633$ and $F = 1.092$, respectively, with d.f. = 1/236 in each case). The interaction effect was also insignificant ($F < 1$). This supports the contention that the recall of P and U adjectives will not differ when attributed to fictitious caste in a nonego-involved context. In experiment I, Lampani was seen as a contrasting group to Bengali. Therefore U adjectives were rated to be more intense and were recalled more than P adjectives when ascribed to Lampani. But in the present experiment neither intensity of affect nor recall of P and U adjectives differed when attributed to either Lampani or Kasanda. These results, in combination with the results presented in Table 4, support hypothesis 4 formulated earlier.

Relation of retention of affective materials to the intensity of their affect under conditions of least emotional involvement could be observed by comparing the intensity of affect of recalled and nonrecalled items. Each comparison of mean intensities of affect presented in Table 5 shows quite consistently that the mean intensities of affect of recalled items are higher than the corresponding means of nonrecalled items. However, the differences are nonsignificant. This lack of significant differences presumably results from a relatively fewer number of recalled items as compared to nonrecalled items. In a nonego-involved context, such as in experiment II, the ratio of recalled items to nonrecalled items is much less than what was observed in experiment I under the ego-involved condition (see Table 5). Thus with a reduction in the relative proportion of recalled items to nonrecalled items, the relation of intensity of affect and recall observed in experiment I is less apparent here. Considering all the recall scores for 60 subjects it is, however, noticed that a total of 326 recalls were obtained as against 874 nonrecalled items. The mean intensities of affect for all recalled and all nonrecalled items were calculated by taking polarities of rating disregarding algebraic signs (M = 2.958, SD = 0.929, and M = 2.820, SD = 0.978, respectively). The difference is significant beyond the 0.05 level (t = 2.23). These results support the hypothesis that, irrespective of the context, mean intensities of affect of recalled items will be higher than those of items not recalled. However, such a tendency would be more clearly shown in an ego-involved situation facilitating recall (as in the case of pleasant adjectives when attributed to Bengali and unpleasant adjectives when ascribed to Lampani in experiment I) than in a neutral nonfacilitating recall situation (as in experiment II).

Taft (1954) has suggested a functional approach to explain selective recall of affective material. Recall of experiences is determined by the function they serve for the organism. This explanation, however, he admits, is *ex post facto*, and, therefore, prediction "for any group of Ss in any given circumstances whether positive and negative ego involvement will lead to sensitization or repression" (p. 27) is not possible. Our findings suggest a framework where, from a knowledge of perceived intensity of affect, prediction about the selective recall of affective material is possible.

Intensity of Perceived Affect under Task- and Ego-orientation

Using the typical frame of reference paradigm, the first two experiments demonstrated that the perceived intensity of affect varied as a function of varying degrees of emotional involvement and that such perceived intensity of material determined its learning and retention.

In a third experiment, the generality of the perceived intensity of affect hypothesis was tested in an experimental framework similar to that used by Rosenzweig (1943). In his study, using interruption technique, Rosenzweig (1943) found that under conditions of low stress, subjects recalled more of interrupted than completed tasks. These results were similar to what is commonly known as the Zeigarnik effect (Alper, 1952). Under high stress, however, subjects recalled more of completed than interrupted tasks, confirming expectations based on Freudian repression hypothesis. Task- and ego-orienting instructions were used to produce respectively low and high stress conditions for his subjects. Rosenzweig explained these results by assuming that under task-orientation, subjects were influenced by a need-persistive drive or a tendency to persist in a task till its completion. Such persistence in the task due to the completion tendency resulted in better recall of interrupted than completed tasks. On the other hand, under ego-orientation, the interrupted tasks were perceived as a threat to the ego. Hence, ego-defensive drive was operative, resulting in poor recall of interrupted tasks as compared to completed ones. It was of interest to see how intensity hypothesis can account for these results.

In designing the experiment it was assumed that incompletion of a task is always unpleasant and that completion of it is always pleasant for the individual, irrespective of whether the individual is operating under task- or ego-orientation. Empirical evidences from various sources (Mandler, 1964) seem to support the above assumption. Yamaguchi (1965) also reports an experiment where, on the whole, completed and incompleted tasks were perceived as pleasant and unpleasant respectively. Moreover, the assumption can always be tested by simply asking the individual to rate his experience with interrupted and completed tasks on a pleasant-unpleasant scale. The usual procedure in experiments using interruption task method is to present the subject with some problems. He is allowed some time to solve each of them. He is not aware when he is going to be interrupted. If the subject is at all involved in the experiment, irrespective of the task- or ego-orienting instructions, he is bound to experience a personal success with completion of a task and a personal failure with its interruption. Task- and ego-orientations only provide two levels (low and high) of emotional involvement for the subject.

However, in this experiment, the subject was not actually interrupted while trying to solve a problem. He was asked to solve each of the problems within 2 minutes and to report his solution when asked by the experimenter after this specified time limit. In the case of half of the puzzles (i.e. 10) his solutions are reported as "wrong" by the experimenter, and yet the correct solutions were never pointed out to the subject. Thus, in case of each of these "unsolved" problems, a sense of incompletion or failure on the part of the subject was induced. In case of the other 10 puzzles, however, the subject's solutions were reported as "right" by the experimenter, thereby inducing in him a sense of completion or success. Thus the procedural technique used in the experiment can be more accurately described as "incompletion" technique rather than "interruption."

Experiment III†

The experiment aimed at finding out how different levels of emotional involvement induced through task- and ego-orientation will have differential effects on perceived intensity of affect associated with one's experience of success and failure, and whether such perceived intensity of affect can adequately explain memory for the success and failure experiences.

Feelings of success and failure were experimentally induced in the subjects under conditions of task- and ego-orienting instructions. The orienting

†The study was previously reported by Dutta and Kanungo (1967). Copyright (1967) by the American Psychological Association. Portions of the previous report are reprinted by permission.

instructions were similar to those used in earlier studies (i.e., Rosenzweig, 1943). The purpose of the task- and the ego-orienting instructions was to create respectively low and high stress or emotional involvement for the subjects. Assuming that the affects of pleasantness and unpleasantness are necessary concomitants of experiences of success and failure, respectively, it was of interest to see the differential effects of such instructions on the perceived intensity of affect of success and failure experiences and their retention. It was thought, for instance, that ego-orienting instructions used in the present study may put the subject on the defensive. This may result in experiencing pleasantness associated with success more intensely than unpleasantness associated with failure because the intensity of experience of failure is minimized and that of success is magnified. On the other hand, particular conditions of task orientation used in this study may make the subject less defensive. Under these conditions the subject may feel unpleasantness due to failure more intensely than pleasantness due to success as he tries to recognize and overcome his failures without caring much for his successes. These considerations lead to the following specific hypotheses:

1. Under task-orientation, unpleasantness of a task due to failure will be perceived as more intense than pleasantness of a task due to success.
2. Under ego-orientation, unpleasantness of a task due to failure will be perceived as less intense than pleasantness of a task due to success.
3. More unpleasant than pleasant tasks will be retained under task-orientation, and more pleasant than unpleasant tasks will be retained under ego-orientation.
4. Mean intensities of perceived affect of the tasks retained will be higher than those of the tasks not retained. This will hold true for both pleasant and unpleasant tasks, irrespective of the orienting instructions.

Method

Materials. Fifty 15 X 15 centimeter colored, irregular abstract designs were prepared. The same colors—red, black, and yellow—were used in each design. An attempt was made to make the designs look as uniform as possible in terms of color, texture, and abstract visual impression. Each design represented a puzzle picture and concealed a very vague and ambiguous figure of an object, animate or inanimate, which the subject had to identify within a specified time period. The figures in the pictures were made ambiguous in order to make the subject depend upon the experimenter's report to know for certain whether he was correct or mistaken in identifying a figure. Even if the subject pointed out the real figure, he could not be absolutely sure of his correctness without asking the experimenter. The following procedure was followed to choose some puzzles of matched difficulty.

All 50 designs were presented as puzzle pictures to 20 judges. While presenting each picture to a judge, the name of the object to be identified in it was mentioned, and 2 minutes were allowed to locate it. Whenever the judge pointed out a figure in the picture other than that which was supposed to represent the named object, he was reported to be wrong and was asked to try again. If the judge failed to identify the correct figure within this 2-minute period, it was pointed out to him by the experimenter. Next, he was asked to rate the degree of difficulty of the puzzle picture on a bipolar nine-point scale extending from extremely easy to extremely difficult, with weights ranging from 1 to 9. The degree of difficulty for each of the puzzle pictures was determined by taking its mean polarity score. Twenty pictures belonging to the middle range of difficulty, that is, falling within a range of 4-6, were selected for the experiment. Each of them concealed a common object such as a car, fish, bird, cup, etc. Care was taken to see that the names of the objects were frequently used words.

Subjects. Sixty graduate students and research workers volunteered to serve as subjects. Each subject was tested individually.

Procedure. Subjects were randomly assigned to two groups of 30 subjects in each. One group (TO) received task-orienting instructions, and the other group (EO) received ego-orienting instructions.

The task-orienting instructions were as follows:

> We ask your cooperation in constructing and standardizing an abstract intelligence test. Several puzzle pictures have been prepared for this purpose. Each picture conceals a specific object which is to be identified by you. From your answers, some of these pictures have to be selected and standardized as final test items. All we want is to check the usability of these pictures for testing purposes by getting your reactions to them.

The ego-orienting instructions were as follows:

> We are going to present to you a very sensitive and reliable puzzle picture test that measures abstract intelligence with a fair degree of accuracy. With this test, we want to know your comparative standing within the selected sample and you will be ranked accordingly in the final analysis. The test consists of several puzzle pictures, each of which conceals a specific object to be identified by you.

After such orientation, each subject of both the groups was given the following instructions regarding the procedure:

> Each picture with the name of the hidden object will be presented to you for 2 minutes. Your task would be to locate that particular object in the picture. You will be given only one chance of giving your answer. Hence, be sure that you point out a particular form representing the said object only after careful consideration of all possible alternatives. This we want to emphasize because more than one form in the picture may appear similar in some way to the named object, and to be correct you have to choose the one that resembles the object most. Please give your answer only when you are asked after the 2-minute inspection period, and not before that. Even if you feel confident that you have

discovered the object, remain silent till you are asked and go on scrutinizing the picture from all possible angles to be doubly sure. If, after carefully scrutinizing the picture for 2 minutes you are not sure of identifying the said object, you must make a guess, however wild it may seem to you. After you give your answer, you will be told whether you have correctly identified the object or not.

Following these instructions, each subject was presented with each of the 20 pictures for 2 minutes for identification of the hidden object. To each picture, the subject responded after a 2-minute period, and then he was only informed whether this solution was correct or wrong. When the subject's solutions were reported to be wrong, the correct solutions were never pointed out to him in order to ensure lack of closure in the subject. After reporting the correctness of a solution, the experimenter then presented to the subject a nine-point bipolar pleasant-unpleasant rating scale with verbally labeled categories. The subject was asked to evaluate on a nine-point scale his experience with the specific task that he had just performed either correctly or incorrectly. Such ratings constituted the degree of affectivity that the subject had experienced with a particular puzzle picture.

The order of presentation of 20 puzzle pictures was randomly varied over 60 subjects. Further, a predetermined pattern of affect was induced in each subject by reporting half of his solutions (10 puzzle pictures) to be correct and the other half (remaining 10 puzzle pictures) to be wrong. In trying to do this, the experimenter took advantage of the abstractness and ambiguity involved in each picture. If, for instance, a particular puzzle meant to be a failure item according to the predetermined pattern, even when the supposedly correct figure was identified by the subject, the experimenter reported it as "wrong." If, however, a puzzle was meant to be a success item according to the predetermined pattern, any figure the subject suggested in the picture was reported to be correct. Thus it was possible for any single puzzle picture to induce a sense of success in half of the subjects and a sense of failure in the other half of the subjects in each group.

After the subjects finished identifying the hidden objects and rating their experiences with each of the 20 pictures, retention tests were administered. Half of the subjects in each group were asked to recall the names of objects concealed in the puzzle pictures. The other half of the subjects in each group were asked to recognize and sort out the puzzle pictures that they had seen before from a pile of 40 pictures. This pile included 20 original puzzle pictures presented to the subjects and another 20 extra puzzle pictures matched as much as possible with the original ones in terms of color, texture, and abstract visual impression. Whether it was recall or recognition, each subject was allowed 5 minutes.

Results

Each subject rated his experience with each of the 10 success puzzles (where success was induced) and 10 failure puzzles (where failure was induced) on a nine-point bipolar pleasant-unpleasant scale. The subject's ratings were transformed into ordinal weights of 0, 1, 2, 3, and 4 for neutral, mild, moderate, strong, and extreme points on the scale, respectively. The weights had a positive value when the subject rated his experience as P and a negative value when the subject rated his experience as U. For each subject, two mean-intensity ratings were calculated: one for the 10 success puzzles and another for 10 failure puzzles. It was noticed that success puzzles were always rated as P and failure puzzles were always rated as U by the subjects. Taking an average of these mean intensities (polarity ratings) in the TO group (n = 30), it was found that the absolute level of perceived unpleasantness associated with failure puzzles was (M = 2.55, SD = 0.576) more intense than perceived pleasantness associated with success puzzles (M = 2.117, SD = 0.624). This difference is significant at the 0.001 level (t = 6.37). Similar averages for the EO group (n = 30) revealed just the reverse pattern. The perceived intensity of pleasant affect associated with success puzzles (M = 2.593, SD = 0.620) was greater than the perceived intensity of unpleasant affect associated with failure puzzles (M = 1.76, SD = 0.733). This difference is also significant at the 0.001 level (t = 6.83). These results support hypotheses 1 and 2.

A 2 X 2 X 2 analysis of variance (Lindquist, 1953, type III design) was performed on the retention scores of the subjects. The three classifications were orientation (task versus ego), retention tests (recall versus recognition), and rated affect (P versus U affect of puzzles). The result of the analysis presented in Table 6 revealed two significant effects. One was the main effect of orientation (F = 8.775, d.f. = 1/56, $p < 0.01$) and the other was the interaction between orientation and affect variables (F = 71.395, d.f. = 1/56, $p < 0.01$). The reasons for obtaining these significant effects can be seen from the total and the mean number of puzzles retained by the subjects under various conditions. An examination of these data as presented in Table 7 indicated that under task-orientation retention was better than under ego-orientation. This can be best explained in terms of the degree of motivational stress experienced by the TO and EO groups. It is quite possible that the EO group faced a more stressful situation, which in turn adversely affected their incidental learning of the puzzle as compared to the TO group. The significant interaction between orientation and affect stemmed from the fact that more U than P puzzles were retained by the TO group and more P than U

Table 6. *Analysis of Variance of Recall Scores*

Source of variation	MS	F
Orientation (O)	19.200	8.755**
Retention tests (RT)	0.824	0.376
O × RT	0.536	0.244
Residual (B)	2.193	
Affect (A)	1.200	1.070
A × O	80.034	71.395**
A × RT	3.343	2.982
A × O × RT	1.630	1.454
Residual (w)	1.121	

** $p < 0.01$, d.f. = 1/56.

Table 7. *Retention of Pleasant and Unpleasant Puzzles*

	TO group			EO group		
	Recall	Recognition	Combined	Recall	Recognition	Combined
P puzzles						
Total score	85	82	167	92	100	192
M	5.667	5.467	5.567	6.133	6.667	6.400
U puzzles						
Total score	108	102	210	73	64	137
M	7.200	6.800	7.000	4.867	4.267	4.567
t	3.992***	3.471**	5.268***	3.296**	6.250***	6.738***

** $p < 0.01$. *** $p < 0.001$.

Note. Each of the differences has been tested by using within-subject error variance. n = 15 for both recall and recognition in TO and EO groups.

puzzles were retained by the EO group. Even when the mean retention scores were calculated separately for recall and recognition tests in each of the groups, the differences still remain statistically significant (see Table 7). These results strongly support hypothesis 3.

It may be pointed out that the pattern of differential retention of P and U puzzles by the two groups (see Table 7) is quite consistent with the pattern of their respective intensities of affect as perceived by the two groups. In the TO group, the U puzzles were rated as more intense and were retained better than the P ones. On the other hand, in the EO group, P puzzles were perceived as more intense and were retained better than the U ones. Such consistency suggests a strong positive relationship between intensity of affect and retention.

The difference between the retention of puzzles rated as P and of those rated as U was found to be nonsignificant (see Table 6). Furthermore, no difference was observed between the two measures of recall ($F = 0.376$, d.f. = 1/56). This might seem to be somewhat unexpected because recognition is generally found to yield a higher retention score than unaided recall. It should be noted, however, that the recognition and recall procedures followed in this experiment make the situation somewhat different. In the recognition test, subjects were asked to select the 20 original puzzles they had been asked to solve from a pile of 40 puzzle pictures. Visually all these pictures were very similar to each other in terms of the colors used and the abstract information they provided. Compared to this recognition test, in the recall test subjects were asked for a free recall of the names of hidden objects in the pictures. These names were frequently used common words of the subjects' language. Thus, it was probably easier for the subjects to recall the common and simple names than to recognize the puzzles from among the very similar abstract designs.

Number of items retained (both recall and recognition measures combined) by both the groups was 706 out of a maximum possible total of 1200 (each of 60 subjects was exposed to 20 puzzles). Thus there were 494 nonretained items. The mean intensity of affect of the retained items calculated from the polarity of ratings on the pleasant-unpleasant scale is 2.548 (SD = 1.051). This mean is significantly higher than the mean of 1.836 (SD = 1.111) calculated for nonretained items ($t = 11.484$, $p < 0.001$). Similar differences are observed between the intensities of affect of retained and nonretained items within P (success) puzzles, as well as within U (failure) puzzles irrespective of whether the subject is in the TO or EO group. Table 8 presents the comparisons between the mean intensities of perceived affect of retained and nonretained items. Such comparisons are shown separately for recall and recognition and for P and U puzzles in each group. For each comparison the mean intensity of affect of retained items is higher than that of nonretained items. Except in one case, the observed differences are statistically significant. The data in Table 8 clearly support hypothesis 4.

Discussion

Retention of success and failure experiences seems to be a function of the perceived intensity of their pleasant and unpleasant affects, respectively. Thus, under specific conditions of task- and ego-orienting instructions as used in the present study, the memory for failure and success experiences can be adequately explained in terms of the perceived intensity of the respective unpleasant and pleasant components associated with them.

Table 8. *Comparisons of Intensities of Affect of Retained and Nonretained Items*

	P puzzles				U puzzles				P and U combined			
	Total	M	SD	*t*	Total	M	SD	*t*	Total	M	SD	*t*
TO group												
Recall												
Retained	85	2.341	1.091	3.173**	108	-2.741	1.161	2.522*	193	2.560	1.158	4.496***
Nonretained	65	1.754	1.137		42	-2.214	1.081		107	1.935	1.137	
Recognition												
Retained	82	2.573	0.898	6.770***	102	-2.716	0.963	3.702***	184	2.652	0.938	7.573***
Nonretained	68	1.632	0.766		48	-2.083	0.997		116	1.819	0.896	
Combined												
Retained	167	2.455	1.072	6.635***	210	-2.724	1.082	4.296***	377	2.605	1.057	8.307***
Nonretained	133	1.692	0.966		90	-2.144	1.040		223	1.874	1.022	
EO group												
Recall												
Retained	92	2.739	0.792	3.066**	73	-2.329	1.060	4.912***	165	2.558	0.942	6.222***
Nonretained	58	2.276	1.030		77	-1.494	1.014		135	1.830	1.092	
Recognition												
Retained	100	2.700	1.005	1.222	64	-1.953	1.138	3.026**	164	2.408	1.121	4.482***
Nonretained	50	2.480	1.082		86	-1.372	1.172		136	1.794	1.238	
Combined												
Retained	192	2.719	0.909	2.983**	137	-2.153	1.114	5.612***	329	2.483	1.038	7.462***
Nonretained	108	2.370	1.060		163	-1.429	1.103		271	1.804	1.180	
TO and EO groups												
Combined												
Retained	359	2.596	0.965	7.143***	347	-2.499	1.129	8.670***	706	2.548	1.051	11.484***
Nonretained	241	1.996	1.064		253	-1.684	1.133		494	1.836	1.111	

* $p < 0.02$. ** $p < 0.01$. *** $p < 0.001$.

Rosenzweig (1943) found that under task-orientation subjects recalled more of interrupted than completed tasks. Under ego-orientation, however, subjects recalled more of the completed than interrupted tasks, confirming expectations based on the Freudian repression hypothesis. Rosenzweig explained these results by assuming that under task-orientation subjects were influenced by a need-persistive drive or a tendency to persist in a task until its completion. It may be noticed that Rosenzweig's findings regarding differential recall of incompleted and completed tasks under two degrees of emotional involvement are consistent with the pattern of retention for success and failure items in the present study. Such consistency leads one to consider the possibility of explaining Rosenzweig's results in terms of intensity hypothesis. One can assume that if a subject is at all involved in an experiment where the interruption technique is used, he is bound to experience a feeling of personal success with the completion of a task and personal failure with its interruption. The affective components of pleasantness and unpleasantness associated with the experiences of personal success and failure, respectively, may account for the recall patterns observed in Rosenzweig's study. In fact, in his study Rosenzweig (1943) observes a concomitant relationship between the completion of a task and success, and also between the incompletion of a task and failure.

The pattern of results obtained under high emotional involvement induced by ego-orienting instruction in the present experiment, and in Rosenzweig's study (1943) are quite consistent with the expectation based on the concept of defensive tendency of an individual. Several formulations of defensive attempts by an individual to reduce the perceived magnitude of a negative affect have been suggested by Peters (Rapaport, 1959, p. 52), Jersild (1931), Festinger (1963), Osgood *et al.* (1957), and others. The operation of defensive response as such, without any reference to the magnitude or intensity of affect, have been used by numerous investigators to explain selective recall of affective experiences, e.g., Brown (1961), Eriksen (1954), Inglis (1960), etc. On the other hand, in a motivational context of low emotional involvements, i.e. when the situation is not too stressful or threatening, "vigilant" rather than defensive response on the part of an individual has been postulated by many investigators (Brown and Yandell, 1966; Bruner and Postman, 1949; Taft, 1954).

Thus, it may be suggested, at least on a hypothetical level, that other things remaining constant, in a defensive situation induced by ego-orienting instructions, an individual tends to perceive pleasant experiences as more intense than unpleasant experiences and consequently stores the pleasant experiences better in his memory. As a result, when tested later, he can recall more of the pleasant experiences than the unpleasant ones. Conversely, in a situation where an individual is quite vigilant and has no need to be defensive, he perceives unpleasant experiences as more intense than pleasant ones. Since the greater the intensity of affect the stronger the impression, he stores unpleasant experiences better in his memory.

Perceived Intensity of Affect and Personality Types

Several studies using the interrupted task method and task- and ego-orienting instructions have suggested that selective learning and retention of affective materials may be a function of personality structure of the individual (e.g. Inglis, 1961). These studies were reviewed in Chapter 2. It was concluded that diverse research literature dealing with the effects of personality type variables does not permit any definite statement regarding the precise relationship between selective learning and retention of pleasant and unpleasant experiences on the one hand, and personality disposition on the other hand. The main reason for this may stem from the lack of clear conceptualization of the nature of many personality variables and also from problems associated with precisely measuring these variables.

One of the studies in the area (Kanungo, 1968) referred to in Chapter 2 dealt with the effects of introversion and extroversion (Eysenck, 1947) on selective memory for pleasant and unpleasant experience. In the following section this study will be described in detail primarily because in the framework of a single experiment the study not only tests the effects of the personality variables of introversion-extroversion, but also brings the perceived intensity hypothesis under test. The study will be referred to as experiment IV.

Experiment IV†

The experiment made use of introverts and extroverts as subjects and tested Eriksen's (1954) suggestion that extroverts would be expected to recall more completed than incompleted tasks while the introverts would behave in the reverse manner. This suggestion was tested under both ego- and task-orientation conditions that provided two degrees of emotional involvements for the subjects. In addition, the experiment was designed to test the

†The study was previously reported by Kanungo (1968). Copyright (1968) by the American Psychological Association. Portions of the report are reprinted by permission.

hypothesis that it is the perceived intensity of affect arising from successes and failures that determines selective retention of completed and interrupted tasks. Thus, for each subject under both task- and ego-orientation conditions, the intensity of affect of retained tasks would be higher than the intensity of affect of nonretained tasks regardless of the quality of affect (pleasant or unpleasant) associated with the tasks. The effects of introversion–extroversion factor, if any, should be noticed, not only in recall but also in subject's rating of pleasantness and unpleasantness of success and failure tasks. Thus, following Eriksen's (1954) suggestion, it is expected that extroverts should perceive pleasant affect due to success more intensely than unpleasantness due to failure. Introverts, on the other hand, should perceive unpleasant affect due to failures more intensely than pleasantness due to success.

Method

Materials. Anagrams of 13 frequently used five-letter words were chosen (Thorndike and Lorge, 1944) as tasks to be solved by subjects. These words are presented in Table 9. For each word, four different patterns of letter arrangements of equal difficulty (Hunter, 1959), namely, 31524, 35142, 52413, and 42531, were prepared. The anagrams were made into four separate series, each comprising the 13 words and containing at least three

Table 9. *Difficulty Indexes and Recall of the Anagrams*

Anagrams solutions	Percent subjects who solved	Percent subjects who recalled	Average time (seconds)
Above	41.67	54.17	42.83
Chair	52.08	58.33	44.88
Dance	45.83	43.75	40.75
Force	45.83	22.92	41.60
Grain	43.75	43.75	42.92
Learn	54.17	43.75	38.29
Light	81.25	41.67	25.15
Metal	22.92	45.83	54.48
Ocean	68.75	62.50	29.17
Plant	66.67	27.08	35.58
Story	54.17	45.83	36.71
Twice	31.25	37.50	44.94
World	85.42	45.83	24.85

Note. For the solution word *ocean* the percentages include subjects who either gave the solution *ocean* or an alternate solution *canoe.* For each column the scores are based on $n = 48$.

examples of each letter pattern. Two easier practice anagrams, DEVLI (devil) and ASUGR (sugar) were also used. Each of the test and practice anagrams was printed on a separate 5 X 3-inch index card. A nine-point bipolar pleasant-unpleasant scale with verbally labeled categories such as extreme, strong, moderate, mild, and neutral was also printed on a 5 X 3-inch index card so that subjects could indicate the degree of affect they experienced with the solving of each task. All cards were placed in a Kardex folder so that the experimenter could expose, in a predetermined random order, first, an anagram for 1 minute to solve, and then the scale to rate the degree of affect associated with the task.

Selection of subjects. The Maudsley Personality Inventory (Eysenck, 1959) was administered to a class of 68 undergraduate students whose ages ranged from 18 to 28 years. The test consists of 48 questionnaire items, half of which are intended to measure extraversion (E-scale) and the other half are intended to measure neuroticism (N-scale). One of three possible responses such as "Yes," "?," or "No" may be given to each item. For instance, the E-scale includes items such as Would you rate yourself as a lively individual? and Are you inclined to keep quiet when out in a social group? An affirmative response to the former item indicates extroversion where a similar response to the latter item indicated introversion. The N-scale includes items such as, Are you inclined to be moody? and Do you often feel disgruntled? Affirmative responses to these items would indicate neuroticism or emotional instability. Out of the 68 subjects who took the test, 24 subjects (14 females and 10 males) who had E-scores of 30 and above (extroverts) and 24 subjects (13 females and 11 males) who had E-scores of 20 and below (introverts) were selected. The extrovert subjects were further divided into two groups of 12 subjects in each matched for their E-scores. The mean E-scores of the two groups were 36.33 (SD = 3.86) and 36.25 (SD = 5.05). Likewise, introvert subjects were also divided into two matched groups of 12 subjects each, having mean E-scores of 14.58 (SD = 3.86) and 14.25 (SD = 4.95). All the four groups were matched for their scores on the N-scale.

Procedure. All subjects were tested individually. One of the extrovert groups and one of the introvert groups received task-orienting instructions and the other two groups received ego-orienting instructions before the tasks were presented to them. Under the task-orientation the subjects were made to believe that their participation in solving the anagram tasks would help the experimenter in selecting a few anagrams for inclusion in a test battery for future use. Under the ego-orientation, the subjects were made to believe that they were appearing for a test in which they would be solving anagrams, and that the anagram test was a very sensitive and reliable measure of their problem-solving ability.

After the orientation, all subjects were given further instructions to solve each anagram as fast as possible within a maximum period of 1 minute. They were told that in the case of failures they would be provided with the solution word, and that after their experience with each anagram they would be required to indicate their feelings (the degree of pleasantness or unpleasantness) associated with the task of solving the anagram (not the solution word as such) on a pleasant-unpleasant scale.

Following these instructions, the subjects were presented with the two practice anagrams one after the other from the Kardex folder, and then rated each task on the pleasant-unpleasant scale after solving it. This was done to ensure that subjects followed the instructions properly. Each subject was then presented with a series of 13 test anagrams from the Kardex folder in a random order. An anagram was exposed to the subject, and if he solved it within 1 minute the time was noted. Then the subject was asked to rate his experience on the nine-point scale. If he failed to solve within a minute, he was told the solution, and was then presented with the nine-point scale to rate his experience. This procedure was followed for each of the 13 anagrams in a series. Since the same 13 anagrams were made into four separate series (containing at least three examples of each letter pattern), each series was presented to three subjects in each of the four groups. Approximately 1 minute after the subject had completed the procedure described above for all 13 anagrams he was asked to recall and write down the solution words of both the tasks which he solved as well as the tasks which he failed to solve in any order he wished.

Results

There were 13 anagrams and 48 subjects, making a total of 624 tasks. Of this total, 333 (53.36%) were solved and 275 (44.07%) were recalled. In order to test whether the difficulty of a task was related to its recall, two separate indexes of task difficulty—solution index and time index—were first calculated. The solution index was calculated by taking the percentage of subjects solving each of the 13 tasks, and the time index was calculated by taking an average of the time spent by the subjects on each task. Each of these two indexes were then correlated with the task recallability as expressed in terms of percentages of subjects recalling each task. The rank correlations between task recall and solution index (n = 13) was 0.08, and between task recall and time index (n = 13), was 0.02. These indexes are presented in Table 9. It seems, then, that the possible effects of variables such as amount of time spent on the tasks or the ease of solving the tasks did not seriously confound the results of the study.

Task performance. A 2 × 2 analysis of variance was performed on the number of tasks solved by each subject to determine whether introverts and extroverts under task- and ego-orienting conditions differ in their task performance. The interaction between the personality variable (introverts and extroverts) and the orientation variable (task and ego) was significant (F = 8.7, d.f. = 1/44, $p < 0.01$). Examination of these data revealed that introverts performed better under ego-orientation (M = 8.33) than under task-orientation (M = 6.67); and extroverts performed better under task-orientation (M = 7.33) than under ego-orientation (M = 5.42). In both the cases of introverts and extroverts the mean differences are significant beyond the 0.05 level (t = 2.24 and 2.58, respectively). It may be noted that extroverts are worse in performance than introverts only under ego-orientation (t = 3.93, $p < 0.001$), while under task-orientation they are as good as introverts (t = 0.89). None of the main effects was significant.

When asked to recall as many of the 13 anagram solutions as he could, each subject could recall some solutions which he had solved himself (success tasks), and some which he has failed to solve until prompted by the experimenter (failure tasks). Thus the total number of tasks (success and failure combined) recalled constituted his recall performance. A two-way analysis of variance was performed on these total recall scores of each subject to see whether introverts and extroverts differed in their recall performance under both task- and ego-orientations. A significant interaction effect between personality and orientation variables was obtained (F = 4.11, d.f. = 1/44, $p <$ 0.05). Observation of the data revealed that extroverts recalled better under task-orientation (M = 6.33) than under ego-orientation (M = 4.83), a difference which is significant beyond the 0.05 level (t = 2.24). Introverts, on the other hand, showed an opposite (M = 5.67 and 6.08 under task- and ego-orientations, respectively) but not a significant trend. The main effects were again not significant.

Selective recall for success and failure tasks. One main purpose of the experiment was to relate a subject's personality to his differential recall for success and failure tasks under task- and ego-orientations. To achieve this for each subject, the number of success and failure tasks recalled were transformed into percentages by using the following formula: number of success (or failure) tasks recalled multiplied by 100 and then divided by the total number of success (or failure) tasks. A 2 × 2 × 2 analysis of variance

(Lindquist, 1953; type III design) was performed on these recall percentage scores. The three classifications were personality, orientation, and tasks (success and failure). The result of the analysis presented in Table 10 shows that while the two main effects of personality and orientations were not significant, their interaction was ($F = 4.54$, $p < 0.05$). These results were already suggested by the previous analysis of total number of recall scores. The only significant main effect was that for tasks ($F = 12.93, p < 0.01$). The mean percentage of recall scores presented in Table 11 reveals that failure tasks were recalled better than success tasks. This was true for both introverts as well as extroverts since no significant interaction effect between the task and personality variables was observed. A significant interaction between task and orientation ($F = 4.42$, $p < 0.05$) stemmed from the fact that under task-orientation, but not under ego-orientation, a significantly greater percentage of failure tasks than success tasks were recalled. The task-orientation differences are significant in the case of both introverts ($t = 2.61$, $p < 0.02$) and extroverts ($t = 3.09$, $p < 0.01$), as can be seen from the data given in Table 11. Similar comparisons under the ego-orientation reveal only nonsignificant differences. It may also be observed that (see Table 11) extroverts' recall of failure tasks was significantly less under ego-orientation than under task-orientation ($t = 3.12, p < 0.01$). The earlier observation that the total recall scores of extroverts were significantly less under ego-orientation than under task-orientation is, therefore, due to a significant drop in the recall of failure tasks alone.

Perceived intensity of task affect. Each subject rated each of the success and failure tasks on a nine-point bipolar pleasant-unpleasant scale. The subject's ratings were transformed into ordinal weights of 0, 1, 2, 3, and 4 for neutral, mild, moderate, strong, and extreme points on the scale, respectively. For each subject, the mean intensity of affect of success and failure tasks was calculated separately. It was noticed that with a very few exceptions success tasks were rated on the pleasant ends and the failure tasks on the unpleasant ends of the scale. The mean affect intensities were analyzed in a manner similar to the analysis of recall scores, using a $2 \times 2 \times 2$ analysis of variance, type III design (Lindquist, 1953). The results are presented in Table 10. Out of the three main effects of orientation, personality, and tasks, only the latter two were significant (see Table 10). The affect arising from failure tasks was rated as more intense (M = 1.98) than the affect produced by success tasks (M = 1.39); and the ratings by introverts of the intensities of their experience with the tasks (M = 1.92) was higher than extroverts' ratings (M = 1.44).

Table 10. *Analysis of Variance for the Recall and the Intensity of Affect Ratings of Success and Failure Tasks*

Source of variation	Recall		Affectivity ratings	
	MS	*F*	MS	*F*
Orientation (A)	506.967	1.19	1.865	1.32
Personality (B)	24.614	<1	5.931	4.20*
A × B	1935.817	4.54*	3.352	2.37
Residual (b)	426.724		1.413	
Tasks (C)	6033.62	12.93**	8.616	26.51**
A × C	2062.111	4.42*	.049	<1
B × C	156.596	<1	.056	<1
A × B × C	529.831	1.14	.059	<1
Residual (w)	466.749		.325	

* $p < 0.05$, d.f. = 1/44. ** $p < 0.01$, d.f. = 1/44.

Table 11. *Mean Percentages of Recall of Success and Failure Tasks*

Group	Success	Failure	*t*
Introverts			
EO	42.41	56.25	1.57
TO	33.46	56.44	2.61*
t	1.01	0.02	
Extroverts			
EO	39.67	39.00	0.08
TO	39.28	66.55	3.09**
t	0.04	3.12**	

* $p < 0.02$ (2-tailed test). ** $p < 0.01$ (2-tailed test).

Intensity of affect and recall. The mean intensities of affect of recalled and nonrecalled tasks were calculated for each subject in order to see if task recall was associated with intensity of affect. Comparisons between the intensities of affect of recalled and nonrecalled tasks are presented in Table 12. There was a significant difference between the mean intensity ratings of recalled and nonrecalled tasks for all the 48 subjects ($t = 2.47$, d.f. = 47), suggesting the recalled tasks had generally given rise to more intense affect than had the nonrecalled tasks. However, this difference is more clearly observed under ego-orientation ($t = 2.49$, d.f. = 23) than under task-orientation ($t = 0.87$, d.f. = 23), and is more clearly noticeable in the case of extroverts ($t = 2.00$, d.f. = 23) than in the case of introverts ($t = 1.53$, d.f. = 23).

Table 12. *Intensity of Affect of Recalled and Nonrecalled Tasks*

Group	Recalled tasks		Nonrecalled tasks		
	M	SD	M	SD	t
EO[(a)]	2.03	0.76	1.68	0.80	2.49***
TO[(a)]	1.56	1.12	1.46	1.10	0.87
Extroverts[(a)]	1.56	0.90	1.34	0.90	2.00**
Introverts[(a)]	2.03	1.01	1.80	0.99	1.53*
All subjects combined[(b)]	1.79	0.99	1.57	0.62	2.47***
Success tasks[(b)]	1.33	1.02	1.33	0.84	0.04
Failure tasks[(b)]	1.91	1.20	1.76	1.27	2.23**

[(a)] $n = 24$.
[(b)] $n = 48$.
* $p < 0.10$ (1-tailed test). ** $p < 0.025$ (1-tailed test). *** $p < 0.01$ (1-tailed test).

For each subject, comparisons were also made between the mean intensities of affect of success tasks recalled and success tasks not recalled, and between the mean intensity of failure tasks recalled and failure tasks not recalled. Table 12 shows that the intensity ratings of recalled tasks are higher than that of nonrecalled tasks only in the case of failure tasks ($t = 2.23$, d.f. = 47). In the case of success tasks, on the other hand, the mean intensity ratings of recalled and nonrecalled tasks do not differ ($t = 0.04$, d.f. = 47).

Discussion

The present results do not agree with the prediction that extroverts would recall more success than failure tasks and introverts would recall more failure than success tasks. Both introverts and extroverts recalled more failure than success tasks, as would be suggested by the nonsignificant interaction between task and personality variables (see Table 10). This tendency, however, was mainly observed under task-orientation (see Table 11), and thus confirms the findings of Zeigarnik (1938). Under ego-orientation there was no significant difference between the recall of failure and success tasks in the case of both introverts and extroverts. This is contrary to Rosenzweig's (1943) observation that more success than failure tasks are recalled under ego-orientation. Such a recall pattern, however, depends upon the degree of ego-threat created by the instructions. In the present study the ego-orienting instructions, while causing relatively greater emotional involvement in the subjects than did the task-orienting instructions, may not have been sufficiently threatening to their egos.

There was some evidence to suggest that the introversion-extroversion dimension may be related to performance measures such as task solution, total recall, and perceived intensity of affect. The task performance and total recall of the extroverts was always worse under the ego-orientation than under the task-orientation. The reverse pattern was noticed in the case of introverts. The extroverts might have been more inclined to preserve or defend a favorable self-image than the introverts. When tested under situations involving self-evaluation, they displayed a denial reaction to anxiety arousal. Their low recall of the failure tasks under ego-orientation clearly suggests that such a denial process may have been in operation. The better performance of the introverts under the ego-orienting condition can be explained by their less defensive, but more sensitive or receptive nature. Introverts are presumably less inclined to defend their self-image, but at the same time are more sensitive to their environment (Franks, 1961). Thus, higher sensitivity or receptivity to experimental instructions may spur the introverts on to better performance under ego-orientation. Such sensitivity in the introverts might also explain why they experienced the task affect relatively more intensely than did the extroverts. The relatively weak affect experienced by extroverts after each task may reflect either their defensiveness (they deny feeling upset) or their insensitiveness (they show an "I don't care" attitude), or both.

The data presented in Table 12 show that the tasks generating more intense affect tend to be recalled better. This gives some support to the intensity hypothesis. However, the affectivity ratings of tasks do not always parallel the recall of those tasks. For instance, under task-orientation or in the case of success tasks the intensity of affect seems unrelated to retention. It could be that the subjects were less emotionally involved under task-orientation than under ego-orientation and, therefore, they experienced more tasks as neutral in affect. Likewise, most of the success tasks tended to produce neutral affect as compared to the more intensely experienced failure tasks (see Table 10). A large number of such neutral ratings might have obscured the relation between the perceived intensity of affect and recall under these specific conditions. This suggests that under conditions in which stimulus materials are experienced as more or less neutral, in affect one would fail to observe the direct relationship between intensity of affect and retention proposed by the intensity hypothesis.

In conclusion, it may be mentioned that all the preceding four experiments support the notion that in general, intensity of an affective experience as perceived by the individual or a group of individuals, may determine selective learning and retention. An experience that has relatively more intense affect than another seems to create a greater impression on the individual and hence is registered better in the memory store. The experiments strongly suggest that any antecedent variable such as context, ego- or task-orientation instructions, or personality structure, etc., that can influence or bring about changes in the perceived intensity of affect of individuals' experiences is also the variable that indirectly affects selective learning and retention. Because perceived intensity of affect seems to be a crucial moderator variable in determining the nature of selective learning and retention, it is important that research in this area pay more attention to conditions affecting intensities of perceived affect than to individual's orientation, attitudes, values, or personality structures. These latter variables are no doubt important, but their effects on selective learning can be much better understood through studying their effects on perceived intensity of affect variable.

CHAPTER 5

Intensity of Perceived Affect and Retrieval

The selective memory mechanism is generally conceptualized as a three-stage process, namely, registration, storage, and retrieval. In almost all the previous studies on the functional relationship between memory and affective experiences, investigators have manipulated the affective variables at the stage of registration or trace information. The studies reported in Chapter 4 on the intensity hypothesis have also dealt with the problem of how different degrees of emotional involvements influence learning or trace formation, as indexed by recall, of materials of differential affective intensity. Although these studies have indicated a direct functional relationship between the perceived intensity of affective items at the time of their acquisition by the individual and his subsequent recall, they have failed to explain how either the storage mechanism or the retrieval mechanism might be influenced by manipulation of affective variables. This chapter concerns itself with the problem of determining the nature of the latter phenomenon. As mentioned earlier, both storage and retrieval processes may conceivably be influenced by the manipulation of any affective variable following registration. But since it is extremely hard to make any definite observation, on the basis of recall measure, regarding the effect of such manipulation on the storage mechanism, the hypotheses as well as the inferences made in this chapter strictly relate the effects on retrieval process and not on storage. Thus the chapter merely aims at determining the relationship between the perceived intensity of affective materials and their retrieval as indexed by recall. Methodologically, the effect of the variable of perceived affect, manipulated following registration and before retrieval, was studied in an immediate memory context.

Three separate experiments were conducted to verify a series of hypotheses related to the problem. The purpose of the first two experiments was to determine the direction as well as the magnitude of variations in the perceived intensity of affective experiences and their retrieval as affected by

(a) high and low emotional involvement induced at the time of registration or trace formation, and (b) introduction of new information meant to induce changes in an individual's emotional involvement after registration and before retrieval. The objective of the third experiment was to study how recall of items presented to individuals at the time of registration in an emotionally neutral context would be affected when an affective frame relevant to those items was introduced during the interval between registration and retrieval. Thus, individuals were exposed to the items in an emotionally neutral context. Following this, an emotionally relevant context to the items already registered by individuals was introduced. Depending upon the experimental group, the new information was meant to introduce a specific referent or context to the items to which individuals had either a positive or favorable attitude, or a negative or unfavorable attitude, or a neutral or indifferent attitude. Following the introduction of such an informational frame, individuals were asked to recall the items. Thus, the third experiment concerned itself with studying the effect of manipulation of affective variables interpolated between registration and retrieval directly on retrieval.

EXPERIMENT V†

The design and method adopted in this experiment were essentially the same as followed in experiment I described in Chapter 4. The major variation introduced in the present study involved the manipulation of the variable of emotional involvement after registration and before retrieval through "reversal" information. At the initial stage, individual subjects in each experimental group were exposed to two sets of adjectives attributed to their own group and a rival group respectively (or to two affectively neutral groups as the case may be). Following this exposure, however, subjects were informed orally that due to a mistake on the part of the experimenter, the two sets of attributes as applied to the two groups had been reversed. This technique of reversing the affective context of the initial stage of registration by introducing new information immediately before retrieval has been used by Weiner (1968) to study the effect of such manipulation on the retrieval mechanism. The data presented by him clearly show that, at least in the case of motivated forgetting, the retrieval mechanism is affected by a reversed information interpolated between registration and retrieval.

†Some of the results of studies mentioned in this chapter were previously reported by Dutta *et al.* (1972). Copyright (1972) by the American Psychological Association. Portions of the previous report are reprinted by permission.

The specific set of hypotheses tested by the experiment is stated below. The first three hypotheses relating changes in perceived intensity of affect of adjectives were derived from congruity principles (Osgood and Tannenbaum, 1955) as well as in terms of the concept of reduction of cognitive dissonance (Festinger, 1963). The first hypothesis, however, was merely a replication of one of the hypotheses supported by the findings of experiment I described in Chapter 1. The last two hypotheses regarding the relationship between affective intensity and retrieval followed directly from the previous findings on the relationship between affective intensity and selective learning and retention.

1. At the time of initial exposure or registration, the intensity of affect of the pleasant adjectives will be perceived as greater than that of the unpleasant adjectives when ascribed to one's own group. On the other hand, the perceived intensity of affect of the unpleasant adjectives will be greater than that of the pleasant adjectives when ascribed to a group considered to be competitors or rivals by subjects.

2. After the introduction of the "reversal" information during storage phase, the affective intensities will undergo changes that are consonant with the new information. Thus, within the set of adjectives originally attributed to one's own group, the pleasant adjectives will now be perceived by subjects as less intense than the unpleasant ones. On the other hand, among the adjectives originally ascribed to the rival or competitive group, the unpleasant adjectives will now be perceived as less intense than the pleasant ones.

3. When adjectives are attributed to two affectively neutral and unfamiliar socio-linguistic groups, there will be no difference between the affective intensity of the pleasant and that of the unpleasant adjectives either before or after the introduction of the "reversal" information.

4. Recall will be directly determined by the intensity of affect as perceived by the subjects immediately before retrieval. Thus, (a) more pleasant than unpleasant adjectives will be recalled when attributed to one's own group, and more unpleasant than pleasant adjectives will be recalled when attributed to a rival or competitor; (b) following "reversal" information, however, more unpleasant than pleasant adjectives as *originally attributed* to one's own group, and more pleasant than unpleasant as *originally attributed* to the rival group will be recalled by the subjects; (c) there will be no difference between the recall of pleasant and that of unpleasant adjectives when these are attributed to two neutral and unfamiliar groups, even after the introduction of the "reversal" information.

5. In terms of perceived affective intensity as measured by subjects'

ratings immediately prior to retrieval, the mean intensity of affect of the adjectives recalled will be higher than that of the adjectives not recalled. This will hold true for both pleasant and unpleasant adjectives, and regardless of the context in which they are presented.

Method

Subjects. An attitude-toward-French-Canadians scale (Dutta *et al.*, 1969) was used to select 120 English-Canadian students showing relatively unfavorable attitudes toward French-Canadians. The rationale for selecting English-Canadian subjects showing relatively unfavorable attitudes toward the French-Canadians was to ensure high emotional involvement on the part of the subjects in the context of the experiment. It was expected that in terms of greater identification with their own group and relative antipathy towards a "rival" group, the English-Canadians would respond to the affective materials (i.e., comparative reports on English- and French-Canadian characteristics) with a high degree of involvement. All the students were taking undergraduate courses at Dalhousie University, Halifax, Nova Scotia, at the time of the study. First, a preliminary sample of over 150 students was selected from a total of 304 on the basis of a specific score criterion, i.e., all scores below the neutral point on the attitude scale, and then from within this sample a group of 120 who volunteered to serve as subjects was finally selected for the study. Precautions were taken to ensure that the subjects used in the experiment did not have any reason to suspect a connection between the attitude questionnaire study and the final experiment. A period of almost 6 months intervened between the administering of the attitude scale on a group of 304 students and the experiment conducted on a group of 120 subjects selected from this population. Moreover, the attitude scale was administered by persons who did not have anything to do with the experiment. These precautions were necessary in order to maintain the credibility of some supposedly authentic research reports used in the experiment referring to "typical" character traits of both English-Canadians and French-Canadians as two distinct socio-linguistic groups, and measures were taken to keep the subjects unaware of the basis of their selection for the experiment. The group comprised 70 females and 50 males with a mean age of 20.09 years.

Materials. Twenty-five pleasant and 25 unpleasant adjectives were given to 50 judges who were asked to rate each of these adjectives on a nine-point bipolar pleasant-unpleasant scale as well as a seven-point unipolar scale for frequency of usage. In the case of the former scale, the judges' ratings were transformed into ordinal weights of 0, 1, 2, 3, and 4 for neutral, mild, moderate, strong, and extreme points on the scale, respectively. The weights had a positive value when the judges rated an adjective as pleasant and a negative value when the judges rated an adjective as unpleasant. In the case of the unipolar frequency scale, verbally labeled categories ranging from extremely low frequency to extremely high frequency were converted into ordinal weights extending from 1 to 7, respectively. Ten moderately pleasant and 10 moderately unpleasant adjectives were selected for the final experiment on the basis of the judges' ratings. All the adjectives were matched in terms of the judges' ratings for their frequency of usage. In addition, steps were taken to ensure the comparability of the adjectives in terms of their recall difficulty or ease, i.e., a free-recall learning situation was employed. Each adjective was printed on a 3 X 5 index card. Twenty undergraduate students were used as subjects. Each card was shown to each of the subjects for 5 seconds, turned over, and followed by the next card. For each subject a different random order of presentation of the 20 cards was followed. At the end of the presentation of the whole series, the subject was asked to write down as many adjectives as he could freely recall regardless of their order of presentation. Thus, recall frequency or retention index of each adjective in free-recall situation calculated on the basis of this simple procedure was also taken into consideration. Finally, two sets of 10 adjectives, each consisting of five pleasant and five unpleasant, were prepared on the basis of the following criteria: (a) the pleasant and the unpleasant adjectives within each set were matched in terms of mean intensity and frequency ratings as well as their mean retention index; (b) the pleasant and the unpleasant adjectives in each set were matched with corresponding adjectives in the other set in terms of the above indices. The two sets of adjectives with their intensity and frequency ratings as well as their recall indices are presented in Table 13.

Next, two different reports, each incorporating all these 20 adjectives (i.e., two sets of 10 each) were prepared. To make the subjects believe in the authenticity of the reports they were presented to subjects in the form of research abstracts. The first report (R_1) contained at the top the following reference:

> BECK, S. H., and GRAHAM, M. L., A comparative study of two Canadian socio-linguistic groups: differences in traits and cultural norms, *International Bureau of Ethnic Research Bulletin* 5, 123 (1965) (abstract).

This heading was followed by a short introductory paragraph as follows:

> The typical socio-cultural characteristics of two linguistic groups in Canada, namely, the English-Canadians and the French-Canadians have been studied from a comparative standpoint. The sample of English-speaking people has been drawn

Table 13. *Two Sets of Pleasant and Unpleasant Adjectives with their Rated Intensity of Affect, Frequency of Usage, and Recall Frequency*

P Adjectives	Mean intensity of affect (n = 50)	Mean frequency of use (n = 50)	Proportion of recall frequency (n = 20)	U adjectives	Mean intensity of affect (n = 50)	Mean frequency of use (n = 50)	Proportion of recall frequency (n = 20)
SET 1							
Confident	1.74	4.98	0.40	Rude	−2.12	4.50	0.53
Independent	1.88	4.86	0.53	Dull	−1.92	5.30	0.53
Dependable	2.40	4.86	0.40	Stupid	−2.20	5.80	0.53
Helpful	2.02	5.26	0.47	Mean	−2.20	5.06	0.53
Affectionate	2.04	4.70	0.47	Lazy	−1.92	5.42	0.33
Mean	2.02	4.93	0.45	Mean	−2.07	5.22	0.49
SET 2							
Warm	1.92	5.50	0.47	Weak	−1.74	5.34	0.47
Cheerful	2.04	5.08	0.40	Unreliable	−2.48	4.52	0.40
Lively	1.72	5.02	0.53	Selfish	−2.52	4.50	0.40
Intelligent	2.32	5.88	0.40	Dirty	−2.06	5.62	0.47
Gentle	2.02	4.54	0.40	Immoral	−1.66	4.58	0.40
Mean	2.00	5.20	0.44	Mean	−2.09	4.91	0.42

from the Maritime Provinces and that of the French-speaking people from Quebec. The major traits which, in general, have been found to characterize each of these two groups are summarized below.

This passage was followed by a list of five pleasant and five unpleasant adjectives headed "English-Canadians" and another list of five pleasant and five unpleasant adjectives headed "French-Canadians". An example is reproduced below:

English-Canadians	**French-Canadians**
Confident	Cheerful
Rude	Lively
Mean	Selfish
Independent	Warm
Affectionate	Dirty
Dull	Immoral
Helpful	Intelligent
Lazy	Weak
Stupid	Unreliable
Dependable	Gentle

The second report (R_2) had the same introduction and content except that in the reference heading the phrase "two Canadian socio-linguistic groups" was replaced by "two Asiatic national groups", and in the text of the abstract the phrase "two linguistic groups in Canada, namely, the English-Canadians and the French-Canadians", was replaced by "two national groups in Asia, namely, Sikkimese and Bhutanese (residents of two small Asiatic states, Sikkim and Bhutan, respectively)".

In order to achieve a counter-balancing design, two different forms of each of the reports were prepared. In the one form of the first report, set 1 adjectives were ascribed to the English-Canadians and set 2 adjectives to the French-Canadians. In the other form, however, the two sets of adjectives were interchanged with respect to the two groups; otherwise the two forms of the report were identical. The same principle was followed for the second report.

Two pairs of booklets were prepared in order to obtain evaluative ratings from the subjects. One pair corresponded to the two forms of R_1 and the other corresponded to the two forms of R_2. In each booklet, all the 20 adjectives ascribed to two groups in the corresponding report were present. By the side of each adjective there appeared the name of the group to specify to whom the adjective was ascribed in the report. Every adjective in a booklet appeared three times to be rated on *three bipolar nine-point scales,* namely, pleasant-unpleasant, good-bad, and favorable-unfavorable. The bipolar scales were printed below each adjective with verbally labeled categories such as, extreme, strong, moderate, mild, and neutral. Thus for each subject each adjective that appeared in the report also appeared three times associated with either English-Canadians or French-Canadians (or, either Sikkimese or Bhutanese, as the case may be) in random sequence. Four different randomly determined sequences of the 20 adjectives were used for each of the three different scales. The respective positive and negative poles were reversed in half of the cases for each scale. Care was also taken to present in varied sequences the three different scales to different subjects by interchanging the order of the sheets bearing the scales.

Procedure and design. The subjects were randomly assigned to five groups of 24 subjects each. The procedure was similar to that used in experiment I, and one group, group I, was used to replicate their findings. The other groups, group II, III, IV, and V, were used in a 2 × 2 factorial design in which there were two levels of emotional involvement and two sequences of experimental stages affecting the order of evaluative rating stage (i.e., rating of adjectives either *before* or *after* the introduction of new affective information).

Each of the five major experimental groups was divided into two subgroups of 12 subjects each so that the two forms of the same report could be presented to two separate subgroups. The two subgroups were treated exactly in the same way for each of the five experimental groups. There were five different stages of the experiment, namely, (a) report-reading stage, (b) initial rating of adjectives in the report, (c) introduction of new information after registration and before retrieval, (d) subsequent rating of adjectives, and (e) recall. Group I had to go through three of these five stages and each of groups II, III, IV, and V, had to go through four of these stages. Each subject was treated individually.

The different stages of the experiment are shown in tabular form in Fig. 1 and are described below:

(a) *Report-reading stage.* During this stage, the first report (R_1) was presented to groups I, II, and III, and the second report (R_2) to groups IV and V. Thus, groups I, II, and III were meant to perceive the materials under high emotional involvement, and groups IV and V under low emotional involvement.

In the case of each group, the report (whether R_1 or R_2) was presented with written instructions that preceded the report. The instructions were as follows:

> We are planning to conduct a small-group research in which we shall be using a set of adjectives that characterize different social groups. However, several features of these adjectives have to be controlled and matched before we can use them in our study. We are seeking your help to achieve this aim. A well-known study on social stereotypes reports a set of adjectives that were found to characterize English-Canadians and French-Canadians [Sikkimese and Bhutanese].

> We might select some of these adjectives for our purpose. Our selection criteria will be based on your evaluation or rating of some of the features of these adjectives.
>
> On the next page, you will find an abstract of the study mentioned above concerning the traits of the English- and the French-Canadian [Sikkimese and Bhutanese] people. Please go through the adjectives as attributed to each of these two socio-linguistic groups very carefully, since you will be required subsequently to rate them.
>
> Thank you.

After the subject finished reading the report it was taken from him. Every subject was allowed approximately 5 minutes to go through this particular stage of the experiment.

(b) *Initial rating of adjectives in the report.* Evaluative rating scales described earlier (also in experiment I) were then given to the subjects in groups I, II, and IV. They were asked to rate the perceived intensity of pleasant or unpleasant affect associated with each of the adjectives attributed to either of the two socio-linguistic groups. Ratings of groups I and II were expected to be influenced by high emotional involvement and the ratings of group IV by low emotional involvement. The subjects were given approximately 12 minutes to rate the adjectives on three different evaluative scales. The time was found to be more than adequate to finish the ratings. At the end of this initial rating stage, the evaluative scales were taken from the subjects.

(c) *Introduction of new information after registration but before retrieval.* Groups II, III, IV, and V were informed that due to a mistake on the part of the experimenter, the two sets of adjectives as attributed to the two socio-linguistic groups in the original research report were interchanged in the typed copy of the abstract presented to them. The procedure adopted to introduce the new "reversal" information was as follows: each subject was run individually in a room fitted with a one-way mirror. A confederate of the experimenter was watching the proceedings through the mirror from the other room in order to be able to make a dramatic entrance into the scene at the right moment. In the case of groups III and V, the confederate entered immediately after the research reports were taken from the subjects, i.e., at the end of the report reading stage; in the case of groups II and IV, however, the confederate entered immediately after the evaluative scales were taken from subjects i.e., at the end of the initial rating stage. Regardless of the timing of his entrance which was dependent upon the treatment sequence for each experimental group, the confederate, along with the experimenter, acted out the same well-rehearsed scenario as precisely and uniformly as possible with every subject. *The scenario:* the confederate rushed into the room,

Group			1. Report reading		2. Initial rating		3. Reversal information	4. Subsequent rating	5. Recall
I	Ia	Report 1	Set 1 (EC)	Set 2 (FC)	Set 1 (EC)	Set 2 (FC)	No	No	Yes
	Ib	Report 1	Set 2 (EC)	Set 1 (FC)	Set 2 (EC)	Set 1 (FC)	No	No	Yes
II	IIa	Report 1	Set 1 (EC)	Set 2 (FC)	Set 1 (EC)	Set 2 (FC)	EC ⇄ FC	No	Yes
	IIb	Report 1	Set 2 (EC)	Set 1 (FC)	Set 2 (EC)	Set 1 (FC)	EC ⇄ FC	No	Yes
III	IIIa	Report 1	Set 1 (EC)	Set 2 (FC)	No		EC ⇄ FC	Set 1 Set 2 (EC) ⇄ (FC)	Yes
	IIIb	Report 1	Set 2 (EC)	Set 1 (FC)	No		EC ⇄ FC	Set 2 Set 1 (EC) ⇄ (FC)	Yes
IV	IVa	Report 2	Set 1 (S)	Set 2 (B)	Set 1 (S)	Set 2 (B)	S ⇄ B	No	Yes
	IVb	Report 2	Set 2 (S)	Set 1 (B)	Set 2 (S)	Set 1 (B)	S ⇄ B	No	Yes
V	Va	Report 2	Set 1 (S)	Set 2 (B)	No		S ⇄ B	Set 1 Set 2 (S) ⇄ (B)	Yes
	Vb	Report 2	Set 2 (S)	Set 1 (B)	No		S ⇄ B	Set 2 Set 1 (S) ⇄ (B)	Yes

Fig. 1. The schematic presentation of the design and five stages of the experiment. n = 24 in each major group and 12 in each subgroup.

Note: EC, FC, S, and B stand for English-Canadians, French-Canadians, Sikkimese, and Bhutanese, respectively.

obviously agitated, with an open journal in his hands (the cover of the journal not visible) and anxiously asked the experimenter to stop the experiment since a "stupid mistake" in the material had suddenly been discovered by him. The conversation and interaction that followed between the experimenter and the confederate were well within the range of the subject's hearing and sight and the subject was very much exposed to what was going on. The confederate conveyed the message to the experimenter that, due to an incredibly stupid oversight, the two sets of adjectives as attributed to the groups in the original research report had been interchanged while preparing the typed copy of the abstract. With adequate amount of annoyance, irritation, and confusion, they compared the abstract and the journal supposedly carrying the original research paper. The subject, of course, was not close enough to be able to see what was in the journal but he got the general idea that the experimenter did find confirmation of a gross mistake in the copy. The experimenter and the confederate then discussed the possibility of stopping the experiment at that point and permitting the subject to leave. But, finally, they decided against it, and, instead, decided that the mistake should be clearly explained to the subject. Both of them agreed that to the extent that the next stages could be carried out on the basis of the corrected information (i.e., the set of adjectives attributed to one socio-linguistic group in the abstract actually referred to the other and vice versa), it would not make much of a difference. It was decided, however, that a new corrected copy of the research abstract had to be prepared before the next subject was asked to participate in the experiment. At this point, the confederate left the room with the journal as well as the research abstract. In an adequately apologetic and embarrassed manner, the experimenter explained the mistake to the subject and asked him to treat the next stages of the experiment on the basis of the correct information whereby the two sets of adjectives were to be interchanged with respect to the two groups. The abstract itself was never again shown to the subject; he was merely informed orally that the abstract previously presented to them was incorrect because of the reversal of the two sets of adjectives with respect to the two groups.

In groups III and V the "reversal" information was introduced prior to the rating stage and in groups II and IV the rating stage preceded the "reversal" information. In the case of the former two groups, it was pointed out to the subjects that the mistake made in the copy of the abstract was also carried over to the rating scales where the adjectives were designated as attributes of either of the two groups not in accordance with the original research report but according to the copy of the "reversed" abstract. Thus subjects were asked to make the necessary correction in their minds while rating the adjectives and to read an adjective designated as "a French-Canadian attribute" as "an English-Canadian attribute" and the one stated as "an English-Canadian attribute" as "a French-Canadian attribute". The same adjustment applied, of course, to "Sikkimese" and "Bhutanese". At the next and final stage of the experiment (i.e., the recall stage), subjects were to give their recall in accordance with the corrected "reversal" information and not according to the incorrect abstract. In the case of groups II and IV, on the other hand, the recall stage immediately followed the introduction of the "reversal" information; thus, all that subjects were required to do was to recall the adjectives as attributed to the two socio-linguistic groups consistent with the reversal information. Since subjects in these two groups had already rated the adjectives prior to the introduction of the reversal information, their ratings, unlike those of groups III and V, were unaffected by the reversal information.

Although fairly elaborate the execution of the whole scenario took about 3-5 minutes only.

(d) *Subsequent rating of adjectives.* Only groups III and V were asked at this stage to rate the adjectives for their affective intensity in a manner similar to the initial ratings of groups II and IV. The rating scales for the former two groups were identical with those for the latter two groups. Thus, the adjectives designated as attributes of the French-Canadians in the rating scale presented to group III were also designated as attributes of the same community in the rating scale presented to group II, and those designated as attributes of the English-Canadians in the former were also specified to be so in the latter. The situation was exactly the same in the case of groups IV and V, where two Asiatic groups, Bhutanese and Sikkimese, were used instead of English- and French-Canadians.

As in the case of the initial rating stage, subjects were allowed approximately 12 minutes to finish their ratings. At the end of this period, the rating scales were taken from the subjects.

(e) *Recall.* Each subject in all five groups was provided with a recall sheet containing two columns—one for each of the socio-linguistic groups mentioned in the report. They were not required to follow any order or sequence but were merely asked to write down as many adjectives as they could recall regardless of their order of appearance in the report itself. The subjects were allowed 5 minutes for recall. The criterion in terms of which each subject's recall score was calculated was that each adjective had to be recalled in association with the socio-linguistic group to which it was attributed. Thus, if an adjective was written by the subject in the wrong column, it was considered as an incorrect response and each subject's correct recall score was composed only of adjectives recalled correctly as attributes of either of the two socio-linguistic groups. This point will be discussed in more detail in the results section.

The experiment was conducted in an incidental learning context; every care was taken to avoid giving any impression to the subject before the final recall stage that he would be asked to recall these adjectives later.†

The four major experimental groups, representing a 2 X 2 factorial design, were thus equivalent in every way except in terms of specific treatment combination. Consequently, any possible variation in the dependent variable, i.e., retrieval mechanism as indexed by *selective patterns of recall* for different groups, could be analyzed and interpreted with direct reference to the manipulation of the independent variables as embodied in the experimental groups.

Finally, in order to see if the procedure appeared authentic to the subjects each subject was interviewed informally at the end of the experimental session. Although the experimenter had a predetermined format incorporating a set of indirect questions in mind, the subject was never given to understand that the experimenter was probing into his reaction to the experiment in a formal and purposeful manner. The discourse was conducted in a conversational spirit. After the experiment was over, the experimenter thanked the subject for his cooperation, asked him whether he liked it, and gradually channeled the discussion that followed in an informal way into certain indirectly framed key questions. The purpose of this probing was twofold; firstly, to find out whether the supposedly authentic research report presented to each subject was believed to be authentic by him; secondly, whether the somewhat dramatic discovery of a mistake in the middle of the experiment appeared as a genuine occurrence to the subject. Anything less than an unequivocal yes to either of these questions would be considered as sufficient ground for rejecting a subject and replacing him by another.

Fortunately (politeness decrees that effectiveness of our deception should be attributed to good fortune rather than to our realistic performance born out of our newly discovered dramatic talent), only five subjects failed to satisfy our criteria of acceptance and were replaced.

†Whereas groups II and IV had a 3-5 minute interval (i.e., reversal information) between last exposure to the adjectives and recall, an interval of only 1 or 2 minutes intervened between last exposure and recall for groups III and V–the groups which received their "reversal" information prior to rating the adjectives. Although this discrepancy might affect the total number of recalls in the two pairs of groups, there are no grounds for expecting it to affect their patterns of recall–the phenomenon of interest here.

Results

Perceived intensity of affect. Under high emotional involvement at the initial rating stage of the experiment, 24 subjects in group I (GI) and GII, rated 10 adjectives (five P and five U) attributed to English-Canadians (EC) and 10 adjectives (five P and five U) attributed to French-Canadians (FC). Thus, each adjective, as an attribute of either of the two socio-linguistic groups, was rated by 24 subjects in each group on three bipolar evaluative scales. As noted earlier, each subject's rating responses were transformed into ordinal weights. The neutral point on the scale was assigned a value of 0, and the mild, moderate, strong, and extreme points were assigned 1, 2, 3, and 4, respectively, with positive signs when the points appeared on the side of the positive pole and with negative signs when they appeared on the side of the negative pole. Each subject's rating score for each adjective was the mean of its intensity ratings over three scales. Each subject had four different mean intensity rating scores (each mean was calculated over five adjectives) corresponding to P adjectives attributed to EC, U to EC, P to FC, and U to FC, respectively.

A three-way analysis was performed on the affective intensity ratings by GI and GII at the initial rating stage. The between-subject classification was GI versus GII. One of the two within subject-treatment classifications was adjectives attributed to EC versus those attributed to FC; the other classification was P versus U adjectives. The results of the analysis are summarized in Table 14. Unpleasant adjectives were rated significantly higher than P adjectives ($F = 7.892$, d.f. = 1/46, $p < 0.01$). The degree to which adjectives were rated as P or U depended, however, on the cultural group to which they were attributed. This is indicated by the presence of a significant interaction between adjectives attributed to EC or FC and P or U affects ($F = 80.382$, d.f. = 1/46, $p < 0.01$). The average mean intensity of affect for each of the four categories in each group (P and U to EC, and P and U to FC), as presented graphically for GI and GII separately in Fig. 2a, clearly shows the basis of such an interaction. In GI, the mean intensity of affect of P adjectives when attributed to EC was found to be greater than that of U adjectives ($t = 5.344$, d.f. = 1/46, $p < 0.001$). When attributed to FC, on the other hand, the mean affective intensity of U adjectives was found to be greater than that of P adjectives ($t = 6.714$, d.f. = 1/46, $p < 0.001$). A similar trend, although not as pronounced, was observed in the case of GII. Here, among the adjectives ascribed to FC, U adjectives were rated to be more intense in affect than P adjectives ($t = 4.714$, d.f. = 1/46, $p < 0.001$). In the case of adjectives ascribed to EC, however, the mean affective intensity of P adjectives was not

Table 14. *Analysis of Variance of Initial Ratings of Affective Intensity (GI and GII)*

Sources of variation	Sums of squares	d.f.	MS	*F*
Between S:	30.139	47		
GI/GII (C)	0.081	1	0.081	0.124
Error (b)	30.058	46	0.653	
Within S:	37.233	144		
EC/FC (A)	0.004	1	0.004	0.027
P/U (B)	1.026	1	1.026	7.892**
A × B	13.665	1	13.665	80.382**
A × C	0.126	1	0.126	0.857
B × C	0.205	1	0.205	1.577
A × B × C	1.619	1	1.619	9.524**
Error (w):	20.588	138		
Error 1 (w)	6.775	46	0.147	
Error 2 (w)	5.998	46	0.130	
Error 3 (w)	7.815	46	0.170	
Total	67.372	191		

** $p < 0.01$.

Table 15. *Comparisons of Intensity of Affect of Pleasant and Unpleasant Adjectives During Initial Rating Stage (GI and GII)*

Group	Adjectives attributed to		Adjectives		*t*
			P	U	
I	EC	M	3.030	−2.394	5.344***
		SD	0.380	0.597	
	FC	M	2.271	−3.070	6.714***
		SD	0.527	0.523	
II	EC	M	2.689	−2.550	1.168
		SD	0.534	0.470	
	FC	M	2.400	−2.961	4.714***
		SD	0.624	0.499	

*** $p < 0.001$.

Note. In Table 15 and in all subsequent tables, minus signs in case of mean affective ratings of U adjectives merely indicate that the values lie on the side of the negative pole of the scale. Comparisons in all cases are made in terms of absolute values of P and U ratings disregarding algebraic signs.

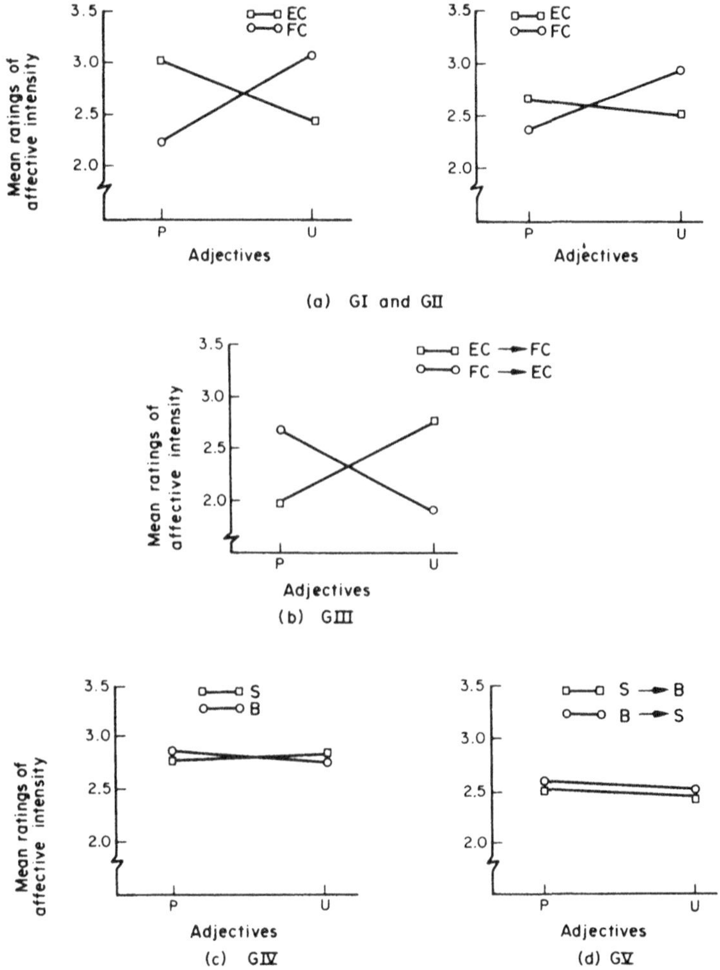

Fig. 2. Affective intensity rating of P and U adjectives (experimentV).

found to be significantly higher than that of U adjectives (t = 1.168, d.f. = 1/46, $p > 0.05$). All the comparisons of mean intensity of affect of P and U adjectives are summarized in Table 15.

The fact that the main effect of the variable of experimental groups (i.e., GI/GII) and its interaction with each of the other two variables (i.e., EC/FC and P/U) were found to be not significant, show the consistency of the rating pattern of GI with that of GII. The significant triple interaction effect (F = 9.524, d.f. = 1/46, $p < 0.01$), however, indicated that the absolute differences between the two P and the two U ratings were different in the two groups. The significant main effect of P versus U affect (F = 7.892, d.f. = 1/46, $p <$ 0.01) resulted from the fact that, on the whole, the affective intensity of U adjectives was greater than that of P adjectives over the two experimental groups. For our purpose, however, the significant interaction between the two main variables, i.e., P versus U adjectives and EC versus FC cultural groups, was most crucial. This interaction, in the case of GI, suggests the confirmation of hypothesis 1. In case of GII, the interaction provides a partial support of hypothesis 1, as already indicated above.

At the subsequent rating stage under high emotional involvement, 24 subjects in GIII rated 10 adjectives (five P and five U) originally attributed to EC but *reported as belonging to FC just before rating;* they also rated 10 adjectives (five P and five U) originally attributed to FC but *reported as belonging to EC before rating.* A threeway (treatment X treatment X subject design) analysis of variance was performed on the mean affective intensity ratings of subjects in GIII. One of the two treatment classifications was adjectives attributed to EC versus those attributed to FC; and the other classification was P versus U adjectives. The results of the analysis presented in Table 16 revealed only one significant effect. This effect involved the interaction between adjectives subsequently attributed to EC or FC and P or U affects (F = 66.374, d.f. = 1/23, $p < 0.01$). The average mean intensity of affect for each of the four categories, as presented graphically in Fig. 2b, shows the nature of this interaction more clearly.

The comparisons of the average mean intensities of P and U affects, following reversal information, revealed that among the adjectives *originally attributed to EC,* U affect was perceived by subjects as more intense than P affect (t = 6.039, d.f. = 23, $p < 0.001$). Conversely, in the case of P and U adjectives *originally attributed to FC,* the affect of the former was found to be more intense than the latter (t = 5.523, d.f. = 23, $p < 0.001$). Thus, the pattern of interaction in this case was found to be in the opposite direction to that observed in the case of the initial ratings reported earlier; the affective

Table 16. *Analysis of Variance of Subsequent Ratings of Affective Intensity (GIII)*

Sources of variation	Sums of squares	d.f.	MS	F
Between (S)	8.275	23		
Within:	25.508	72		
EC → FC/FC → EC (A)	0.261	1	0.261	2.394
P/U (B)	0.026	1	0.026	0.119
A × B	13.142	1	13.142	66.374**
A × S	2.504	23	0.109	
B × S	5.015	23	0.218	
A × B × S	4.560	23	0.198	
Total	33.783	95		

** $p < 0.01$.

Table 17. *Comparisons of Intensity of Affect of Pleasant and Unpleasant Adjectives During Subsequent Rating Stage (GIII)*

Group		Adjectives		t
		P	U	
EC → FC	M	2.002	-2.775	6.039***
	SD	0.512	0.431	
FC → EC	M	2.638	-1.931	5.523***
	SD	0.449	0.492	

*** $p < 0.001$.

intensities of P and U adjectives originally attributed to EC and FC underwent changes in GIII in the predicted direction consistent with the reversal information. Comparison between Fig. 2a and b will make the contrast between the affective intensity *before* reversal information and that *after* reversal information quite obvious. Table 17 summarizes the comparisons of mean affective intensities of P and U adjectives as perceived after reversal information by GIII. The results revealed, as in the case of initial ratings of GI and GII, that the affective intensity of the same adjectives, following reversal information, was also perceived differently depending upon whether they were attributed subsequently to the subject's own or rival group.

To conclude, a comparison of the initial ratings of GI and GII and the subsequent ratings of GIII confirmed the prediction that introduction of the reversal information would reverse the pattern of affective intensity of adjectives consistent with the new information. Hypothesis 2 is thus supported.

GIV and GV rated the affective intensity of adjectives under low emotional involvement, GIV *before* the introduction of reversal information, and GV *after*. A three-way analysis was performed on the initial ratings of the adjectives by GIV. None of the effects analyzed in this case were statistically significant. Similar nonsignificant effects were obtained when an analysis of variance was performed on the subsequent ratings of the adjectives by subjects in GV.

The comparisons between the average mean intensities of affect for GIV and those for GV are presented graphically in Fig. 2c and d, respectively. Figure 2c and d together show clearly the essential similarity between the pattern of affective intensity as revealed by the initial ratings of GIV and that manifested in the subsequent ratings of GV. In each case, the difference between the mean affective intensity of P adjectives and that of U adjectives (regardless of whether they were attributed to the Sikkimese (S) or the Bhutanese (B)) was found to be nonsignificant. When Fig. 2c and d are compared to Fig. 2a and b, respectively, the absence of any significant difference between the intensity of P adjectives and that of U adjectives, regardless of whether they were attributed to two neutral groups before or after the introduction of the reversal information, becomes very striking. The average mean intensities of affect for GIV and GV are summarized separately in Tables 18 and 19 respectively.

The initial ratings of GIV and the subsequent ratings of GV together thus confirm hypothesis 3.

Recall. The recall scores for each group were separately analyzed. In terms of the criterion already stated, each subject's recall score included only those adjectives that were recalled correctly as attributes of either of the two groups. It would also be of interest to treat the recall data disregarding this criterion; thus, all the adjectives correctly recalled, irrespective of whether they were written in the right or wrong column, would constitute the total recall score of each subject. After looking into the recall data, however, an additional analysis on this basis did not seem to be worth while. The subjects in all groups made surprisingly few mistakes in this regard. In most cases, the adjectives correctly recalled were correctly attributed as well, and in none of the groups instances of mistaken shifts exceeded 10% of the correct recalls. It may also be noted here that the study was mainly concerned with determining the pattern or distribution rather than the total number of adjectives recalled by each group. It would be impossible to determine the recall score for each category (i.e., EC or FC, S or B) once the stated criterion of calculating the recall scores for each group is disregarded. For example,

Table 18. *Average Mean Intensities of Affect of Pleasant and Unpleasant Adjectives During Initial Rating Stage (GIV)*

Group		Adjectives P	U
S	M	2.769	-2.789
	SD	0.406	0.406
B	M	2.825	-2.780
	SD	0.424	0.434

Table 19. *Average Mean Intensities of Affect of Pleasant and Unpleasant Adjectives During Subsequent Rating Stage (GV)*

Group		Adjectives P	U
S → B	M	2.564	-2.532
	SD	0.451	0.458
B → S	M	2.600	-2.558
	SD	0.442	0.561

with the exception of the GI condition, the same adjectives were first attributed to one of the cultural groups and then through the reversal information were attributed to the other. Thus, one would not know how to categorize an adjective which, though recalled, was attributed to the wrong group (i.e., not in accordance with the reversal information) by the subject. In order to take that adjective into consideration in determining the recall score of the subject, it would be necessary to categorize the adjective under either of the two socio-cultural groups; and clearly the choice could merely be an arbitrary one. Thus, the wrongly attributed adjectives were disregarded all through the analysis of the recall scores.

A treatment X treatment X subject analysis of variance on the recall scores of GI was performed. The results presented in Table 20 revealed that only the interaction between the two treatments, i.e., EC/FC and P/U, was significant. The basis of this interaction can be seen very clearly in the comparisons between the mean recall scores for the four treatment combinations as

Table 20. *Analysis of Variance of Recall Scores (GI)*

Sources of variation	Sums of squares	d.f.	MS	*F*
Between (S)	25.125	23		
Within:	61.500	72		
EC/FC (A)	0.375	1	0.375	0.775
P/U (B)	0.375	1	0.375	0.775
A × B	22.042	1	22.042	30.785**
A × S	11.125	23	0.484	
B × S	11.125	23	0.484	
A × B × S	16.458	23	0.716	
Total	86.625	95		

** $p < 0.01$.

Table 21. *Comparisons of Pleasant and Unpleasant Recalls Under Two Different Conditions (GI)*

Group		Adjectives		
		P	U	*t*
EC	M	3.792	2.708	4.443***
	SD	0.656	1.043	
FC	M	2.708	3.542	3.418**
	SD	0.752	0.831	

*** $p < 0.001$. ** $p < 0.01$.

graphically presented in Fig. 3a. It was found that the mean recall of P adjectives was higher than that of U adjectives when both were attributed to EC (t = 4.443, d.f. = 23, $p < 0.001$). On the other hand, the mean recall of U adjectives was found to be significantly greater than the mean recall of P adjectives when they both were attributed to FC (t = 3.418, d.f. = 23, $p <$ 0.01). The mean recall score for each of the four categories is presented in Table 21. Finally, it was noted that the pattern of recalls of GI as revealed by Table 21 was quite consistent with the pattern of initial ratings of GI as well as of GII as presented in Table 15. This consistency becomes more apparent when Fig. 2a representing the initial ratings of GI and GII is compared with Fig. 3a, where each of the former very closely resembles the latter. On the one hand, when ascribed to EC, P adjectives were perceived as more intense in affect and were also recalled more frequently than U adjectives. On the other

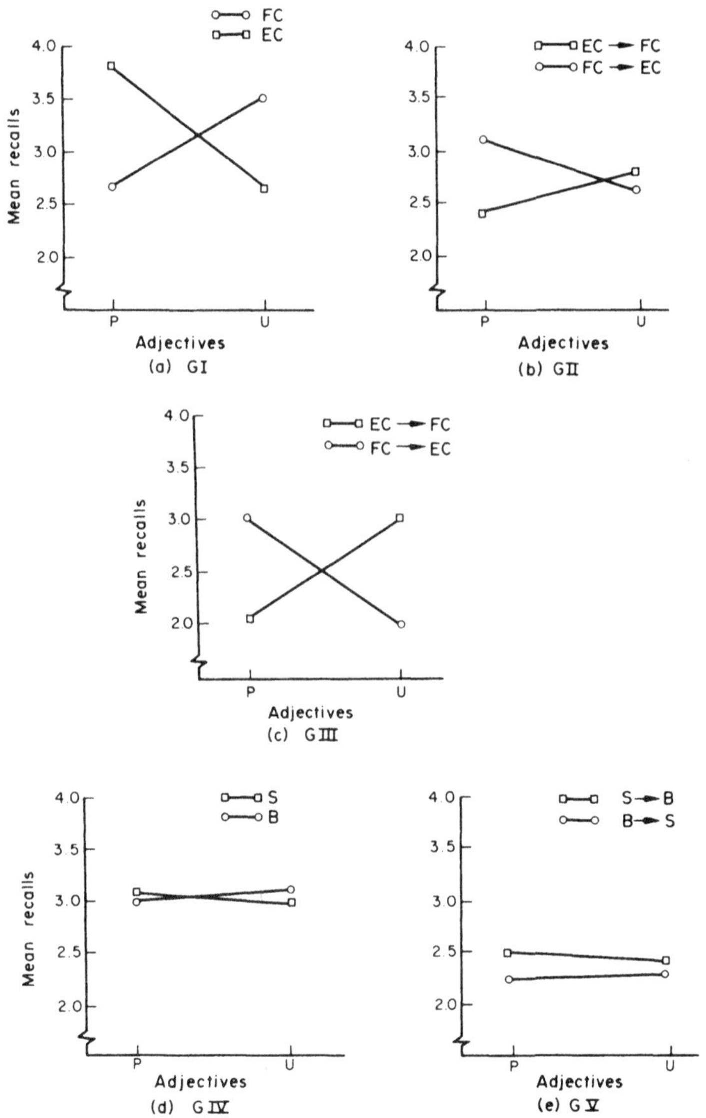

Fig. 3. Selective patterns of recall of P and U adjectives (experiment V).

hand, when ascribed to FC, U adjectives were perceived as more intense and were also recalled to a greater extent than P adjectives. Thus, as hypothesized by the investigator, the recall pattern of GI was found to be in complete accord with the pattern of affective intensity ratings of the adjectives.

Hypothesis 4(a) is thus supported by the observed recall patterns of GI.

An analysis of variance was performed on the recall scores of each of the two groups, GII and GIII, the results of which are summarized in Tables 22 and 23 respectively.

It will be seen that in each case only the interaction between the two treatments was significant. Figure 3b and c clearly show the basis of this

Table 22. *Analysis of Variance of Recall Scores (GII)*

Sources of variation	Sums of squares	d.f.	MS	*F*
Between (S)	62.656	23		
Within:	51.750	72		
EC → FC/FC → EC (A)	1.760	1	1.760	2.316
P/U (B)	0.010	1	0.010	0.019
A × B	5.511	1	5.511	8.598*
A × S	17.490	23	0.760	
B × S	12.240	23	0.532	
A × B × S	14.739	23	0.641	
Total	114.406	95		

* $p < 0.01$.

Table 23. *Analysis of Variance of Recall Scores (GIII)*

Sources of variation	Sums of squares	d.f.	MS	*F*
Between (S)	49.990	23		
Within:	83.750	72		
EC → FC/FC → EC (A)	0.094	1	0.094	0.090
P/U (B)	0.094	1	0.094	0.119
A × B	23.010	1	23.010	29.016*
A × S	24.156	23	1.050	
B × S	18.156	23	0.789	
A × B × S	18.240	23	0.793	
Total	133.740	95		

* $p < 0.01$.

interaction effect in each case. The recall patterns for the two groups were essentially quite similar to each other. In the case of GII (i.e., Fig. 3b), among the adjectives originally attributed to EC and later reported as belonging to FC, U adjectives appeared to be recalled more frequently than P adjectives, although the difference failed to reach the level of statistical significance (t = 1.983, d.f. = 23, $p > 0.05$). On the other hand, among the adjectives originally attributed to FC and later stated to be the characteristics of EC, P adjectives were recalled better than U adjectives (t = 2.164, d.f. = 23, $p <$ 0.05).

What was merely a trend in the pattern of recall by GII was found to be very clear and explicit in the case of GIII (i.e., Fig. 3c). Among the adjectives originally ascribed to EC and later stated as characteristic of FC, the mean recall of U adjectives was found to be greater than that of P adjectives (t = 3.568, d.f. = 23, $p < 0.01$). On the other hand, among the adjectives originally stated to be the attributes of FC and later attributed to EC, P adjectives were recalled better than U adjectives (t = 4.054, d.f. = 23, $p <$ 0.001).

The mean recall scores for GII and GIII are summarized in Tables 24 and 25, respectively.

In summary, following the reversal information, the recall pattern of GIII was found to be in the reverse direction to that of GI. In the case of GII, too, the trend, though not statistically significant, was clearly comparable to the recall pattern of GIII and in the opposite direction to that of GI. Introduction of reversal information not only reversed the pattern of affective intensity, as revealed by the subsequent ratings of GIII (Table 17), but also, in conformity with the reversed pattern of affective intensity, changed the recall patterns of GII and GIII (see Tables 24 and 25, respectively). When Fig. 2b is compared with either of Fig. 3b and c, the consistency between differential affective intensity of the adjectives following reversal information and their differential recall by subjects subsequently will become more obvious. The subjects in GII did not rate the adjectives following the reversal information, and thus, no measure of any change in their affective intensity brought about by such information was available; but the subsequent ratings of GIII did provide us with tangible evidence of a reversal in affective intensity consistent with the new information. This observation, added to the empirical finding that in both groups adjectives were recalled in the same way, leads one to conclude that in GII, too, the perceived intensities of affect had undergone changes following reversal information and influenced their subsequent recall pattern.

Table 24. *Comparisons of Pleasant and Unpleasant Recalls Under Two Different Conditions (GII)*

Group		Adjectives		t
		P	U	
EC → FC	M	2.417	2.875	1.983
	SD	1.138	1.034	
FC → EC	M	3.167	2.667	2.164*
	SD	0.867	1.239	

* $p < 0.05$.

Table 25. *Comparisons of Pleasant and Unpleasant Recalls Under Two Different Conditions (GIII)*

Group		Adjectives		t
		P	U	
EC → FC	M	2.125	3.042	3.568**
	SD	1.154	1.159	
FC → EC	M	3.042	2.000	4.054***
	SD	0.998	1.063	

*** $p < 0.001$. ** $p < 0.01$.

The recall pattern of GIII thus clearly supports hypothesis 4b. In the case of GII, however, the hypothesis is only partially supported by the observed pattern of recall.

Next, the recall scores for the two groups under low emotional involvement, i.e., GIV and GV, were analyzed. The results of the analyses of variance revealed that in each case none of the effects was found to be significant. In particular, the lack of a significant interaction effect in each case could be seen more clearly in Fig. 3d and e, respectively. The absence of such interaction effects in these two groups was in clear contrast with the significant interaction effect observed in the recall scores of each of the earlier three groups under high emotional involvement, namely, GI, GII, and GIII. In the case of GIV and GV, regardless of whether the reversal information was introduced before or after the rating stage, and regardless of whether the adjectives were originally attributed to Sikkimese or Bhutanese and later

Table 26. *Comparisons of Pleasant and Unpleasant Recalls Under Two Different Conditions (GIV)*

Group		Adjectives P	U
S → B	M	3.083	2.958
	SD	1.349	1.460
B → S	M	3.000	3.167
	SD	1.319	1.403

Table 27. *Comparisons of Pleasant and Unpleasant Recalls Under Two Different Conditions (GV)*

Group		Adjectives P	U
S → B	M	2.500	2.417
	SD	1.142	1.501
B → S	M	2.292	2.375
	SD	1.334	1.209

reversed, P and U adjectives were recalled equally well. The mean recall scores of GIV and GV, presented in Tables 26 and 27, respectively, show the comparability of P and U recall in each case. Furthermore, the pattern of recall in the case of each of these two groups was consistent with the pattern of affective intensity of the adjectives as revealed by the initial ratings of GIV as well as the subsequent ratings of GV (see Table 18 and 19).

The consistency between the perceived intensity of affect following reversal information and the subsequent recalls of the two groups under low emotional involvement can be observed more clearly by comparing Fig. 2d and Fig. 3d and e. In this context, the perceived equality between the affective intensity of P and U adjectives, unaffected by any reversal information, was consistent with the observed fact that they were recalled by subjects in both the groups to the same extent under each condition.

Hypothesis 4(c) is thus supported by the recall pattern of each of the two groups, GIV and GV.

Total recall. In view of the apparent variations in total recalls over the four major experimental groups in the 2 X 2 factorial design, a simple two-way analysis of variance was performed on the total recalls of GII, GIII, GIV, and GV. One of the two classifications was high versus low emotional involvement, and the other classification was reversal information after as opposed to reversal information before rating. The results, presented in Table 28, revealed that only the main effect of the variable concerning the reversal information was significant. The mean recall scores for each of the four groups are presented in Table 29. Under both high and low emotional involvement, the group that had its reversal information after rating recalled more adjectives than the group that had its reversal information before rating. This difference reached statistical significance only between the groups with low emotional involvement ($t = 2.524$, d.f. = 92, $p < 0.02$). As noted earlier, the two groups who were exposed to reversal information after rating (GII and

Table 28. *Analysis of Variance of Total Recall Scores (GII, GIII, GIV, and GV)*

Sources of variation	Sums of squares	d.f.	MS	*F*
High versus low emotional involvement (A)	1.260	1	1.260	0.097
Reversal before versus after rating (B)	75.260	1	75.260	5.797*
A X B	17.511	1	17.511	1.349
Error	1194.375	92	12.982	
Total	1288.406	95	1.349	

* $p < 0.05$.

Table 29. *Comparisons of Total Recalls Under Four Treatment Combinations (GII, GIII, GIV, and GV)*

High emotional involvement				Low emotional involvement			
Group	M	SD	*t*	Group	M	SD	*t*
II. Reversal after rating	11.125	3.301		IV. Reversal after rating	12.208	4.243	
			0.882				2.524*
III. Reversal before rating	10.208	2.950		V. Reversal before rating	9.583	3.788	

* $p < 0.02$.

GIV) had a somewhat greater time interval (approximately 3 minutes) between the last exposure to the adjectives and their recall than did the other two groups (GIII and GIV). If the time lag was a significant factor one would expect the latter two groups to recall better than the former; but trend seemed to be in the opposite direction, and this is difficult to interpret. One may argue that where the reversal information was presented to subjects after their last exposure to the adjectives (GII and GIV), the adjectives were already coded by them in terms of two clear-cut category labels. Perhaps all that these subjects had to do was to retrieve the adjectives in terms of their original categories (i.e., EC and FC or S and B, as the case might be) and then transfer the items in one set to the other and vice versa. The subjects who were given the rating scales following reversal information (GIII and GV) had to rate adjectives designated as characterizing EC and FC (or S and B) *not* in accordance with the reversal information, but with the original report. Consequently, they had to read the designations "correctly" by interchanging them with one another and then give their ratings on the basis of such corrections. Conceivably, this process might have created some stress or confusion on the part of subjects and reduced the magnitude of their total recall as compared to those of GII and GIV. The above explanation is admittedly speculative and *ex post facto,* but at this point it is difficult to suggest a more plausible one. One might expect from this explanation that the poorer recall scores of GIII and GV would be produced by the assignment of adjectives to the wrong category. This was not the case. Few category errors were made; in none of the groups did category confusion exceed 10% of the correct recalls.

The absence of any significant effect of the other main variable, i.e., high versus low emotional involvement, on recall should also be noted as somewhat unexpected. It is generally suggested (e.g., Edwards, 1941; Heyer and O'Kelley, 1949; Kanungo and Das, 1960; Levine and Murphy, 1943; Taft, 1954; etc.) that items having high motivational or emotional relevance to an individual are likely to be remembered better by him than those having low motivational relevance. Thus, one would expect that subjects would show better recall for adjectives referring to EC and FC than for adjectives attributed to two unfamiliar Asiatic communities, Sikkimese and Bhutanese. The results clearly show that this was not the case. It is the *kind* of motivational relevance rather than its degree which seems to have influenced the different patterns of recall obtained from subjects in different groups.

Affective intensity and recall. More substantive support for the intensity hypothesis as applicable to retrieval can be found from the test of hypothesis 5.

Comparisons of mean intensities of affect (as perceived immediately before retrieval) of recalled and nonrecalled items for GI, GIII, and GV, have been presented separately in Tables 30, 31, and 32, respectively. It will be observed that in the case of GI (Table 30), a total of 306 recalls was obtained from subjects as against 174 nonrecalled items. The mean intensity of affect of recalled items calculated from the polarity of ratings disregarding algebraic signs was 2.996 (SD = 0.729). This was found to be higher than the mean affective intensity of nonrecalled items (M = 2.157, SD = 0.919). The difference was significant (t = 11.039, d.f. = 478, $p < 0.001$). Comparisons were also made separately for P and U adjectives, and for adjectives attributed to EC and FC. For each comparison, the mean intensity of affect of recalled items was significantly higher than that of nonrecalled items.

Table 31 shows similar comparisons between mean intensities of affect of recalled and nonrecalled items for GIII. Taking all recall scores for subjects, the total number of recalls was found to be 245 as opposed to a total 235 nonrecalled items. As in the case of GI, the mean affective intensity of recalled items (M = 2.723, SD = 0.813) was found to be higher than the mean intensity of affect of nonrecalled items (M = 1.935, SD = 0.898). This difference, too, was significant (t = 10.102, d.f. = 478, $p < 0.001$). Even when broken down into detailed categories, the affective intensity of recalled items was found to be higher than that of the nonrecalled items in each case.

The same comparative analysis of the recalled and nonrecalled items for GV has been presented in Table 32. It will be observed that a total of 230 recalls was obtained as against 250 nonrecalled items. The mean affective intensity of the former was calculated as 2.946 (SD = 0.588) which was higher than the mean affective intensity of the latter (M = 2.220, SD = 0.852). The difference was significant (t = 10.676, d.f. = 478, $p < 0.001$). As in the case of the two previous tables, the breakdown of total recalled as well as nonrecalled items into separate categories consistently confirmed this overall effect. In each case, the mean affective intensity of the recalled items was found to be greater than that of the nonrecalled items at the 0.001 level of significance.

Hypothesis 5 is thus supported by the direct relationship between affective intensity and recall as revealed by the results obtained in the case of each of the three experimental groups, GI, GIII, and GV.

Since subjects in GII and GIV rated the affective intensity of the adjective prior to the reversal information, no such relationship between affect ratings and retrieval was expected in their case. It was inferred, on the basis of the subsequent rating patterns of GIII, that a similar reversal in the pattern of

Table 30. *Comparisons of Intensities of Affect of Recalled and Nonrecalled Items (GI)*

		P				U				P + U			
		n	M	SD	*t*	*n*	M	SD	*t*	*n*	M	SD	*t*
EC	Recalled	91	3.187	0.535	5.055	65	−2.723	0.813	4.626	156	2.994	0.702	7.731
	Nonrecalled	29	2.540	0.754	***	55	−2.006	0.871	***	84	2.190	0.871	***
FC	Recalled	65	2.651	0.685	5.743	85	−3.263	0.702	4.277	150	2.998	0.757	7.786
	Nonrecalled	55	1.824	0.876	***	35	−2.600	0.894	***	90	2.126	0.961	***
Total	Recalled	156	2.964	0.656	8.670	150	−3.029	0.799	6.947	306	2.996	0.729	11.039
	Nonrecalled	84	2.071	0.904	***	90	−2.237	0.927	***	174	2.157	0.919	***

*** $p < 0.001$.

Note: *n* column gives the total number of recalled and nonrecalled items over 24 subjects. Means of combined (P + U) were calculated from the subject's polarity of ratings disregarding algebraic signs.

Table 31. *Comparisons of Intensities of Affect of Recalled and Nonrecalled Items (GIII)*

		P				U				P + U			
		n	M	SD	*t*	*n*	M	SD	*t*	*n*	M	SD	*t*
EC → FC	Recalled	51	2.385	0.862	4.137	73	−3.055	0.684	4.636	124	2.779	0.832	7.345
	Nonrecalled	69	1.719	0.859	***	47	−2.341	0.714	***	116	1.971	0.860	***
FC → EC	Recalled	73	2.923	0.622	5.620	48	−2.272	0.856	3.246	121	2.664	0.793	6.830
	Nonrecalled	47	2.198	0.774	***	72	−1.704	0.976	***	119	1.899	0.934	***
Total	Recalled	124	2.702	0.776	7.443	121	−2.744	0.850	6.793	245	2.723	0.813	10.102
	Nonrecalled	116	1.913	0.859	***	119	−1.956	0.934	***	235	1.935	0.898	***

*** $p < 0.001$.

Note: *n* column gives the total number of recalled or nonrecalled items over 24 subjects. Means of combined (P + U) were calculated from the subject's polarity of ratings disregarding algebraic signs.

Table 32. *Comparisons of Intensities of Affect of Recalled and Nonrecalled Items (GV)*

		P				U				P + U			
		n	M	SD	*t*	*n*	M	SD	*t*	*n*	M	SD	*t*
S → B	Recalled	60	3.000	0.535	6.141	58	−2.286	0.609	4.576	118	2.932	0.577	7.550
	Nonrecalled	60	2.128	0.955	***	62	−2.226	0.869	***	122	2.177	0.915	***
B → S	Recalled	55	2.921	0.577	4.459	57	−3.000	0.613	6.429	112	2.962	0.593	7.714
	Nonrecalled	65	2.328	0.819	***	63	−2.190	0.744	***	128	2.260	0.786	***
Total	Recalled	115	2.962	0.558	7.526	115	−2.930	0.617	7.681	230	2.946	0.588	10.676
	Nonrecalled	125	2.232	0.893	***	125	−2.208	0.808	***	250	2.220	0.852	***

*** $p < 0.001$.

Note: n column gives the total number of recalled or nonrecalled items over 24 subjects. Means of combined (P + U) were calculated from the subject's polarity of ratings disregarding algebraic signs.

Table 33. *Comparisons of Intensities of Affect of Recalled and Nonrecalled Items (GIV)*

		P				U				P + U			
		n	M	SD	*t*	*n*	M	SD	*t*	*n*	M	SD	*t*
S → B	Recalled	74	2.937	0.672	3.237	71	−3.052	0.688	4.852	145	2.993	0.684	5.684
	Nonrecalled	46	2.500	0.780	***	49	−2.408	0.744	***	95	2.453	0.762	***
B → S	Recalled	72	3.042	0.631	4.268	76	−3.062	0.672	5.326	148	3.052	0.654	6.292
	Nonrecalled	48	1.500	0.736	***	44	−2.295	0.882	***	92	2.402	0.816	***
Total	Recalled	146	2.989	0.654	5.315	147	−3.057	0.681	7.163	293	3.023	0.669	8.880
	Nonrecalled	94	2.500	0.758	***	93	−2.355	0.813	***	187	2.428	0.789	***

*** $p < 0.001$.

Note: n column gives the total number of recalled or nonrecalled items over 24 subjects. Means of combined (P + U) were calculated from the subject's polarity of ratings (i.e., initial) disregarding algebraic signs.

affective intensity was brought about in the case of GII and that this reversal would eliminate the relationship that would otherwise exist between ratings and recall. The results were in accordance with this expectation. The mean affect ratings of the 267 adjectives recalled by GII was 2.702 (SD = 0.809); the mean of the 213 nonrecalled items was 2.585 (SD = 0.854). The difference between these two means was not statistically significant ($t = 1.539, p < 0.05$). The failure to obtain a significant difference between the intensity of recalled and that of nonrecalled items, invalidates the assumption that the affective intensities of the adjectives, as revealed by the initial ratings of GII, remained unaffected by the reversal information. Instead, our original inference based primarily on the pattern of recall by GII, that the reversal information did, in fact, bring about changes in initially perceived affective intensity of the adjectives in the predicted directions, seems to be reinforced by the results.

Although GIV, like GII, also rated the adjectives before receiving reversal information, the reversal in attributes between Sikkimese and Bhutanese, being emotionally irrelevant, was not expected to change the affective intensity of the adjectives. Thus, the adjectives recalled by GIV should have received higher affective ratings than adjectives not recalled. Table 33 shows that this expectation was borne out, not only in the total items recalled, but in the separate categories as well. The total number of recalls for GIV was 293 as against a total of 187 nonrecalled items. The mean affective intensity of the recalled items was calculated as 3.023 (SD = 0.669) which was significantly higher than the mean affective intensity (M = 2.428, SD = 0.789) of the nonrecalled items ($t = 8.880, p < 0.001$).

Thus, the results for GIV gave further support to the contention that under the condition of low emotional involvement, the introduction of a reversal information does not produce the effect observed under the condition of high emotional involvement.

Experiment VI

The results of experiment V confirmed each of the hypotheses, and thus generally showed the effectiveness of an affective variable, manipulated subsequent to registration and prior to retrieval, in influencing the perceived intensity of affective materials and their consequent retrieval. Before discussing the implications of the results obtained in experiment V, experiment VI will be introduced at this point since the latter was an exact replication of the former except in terms of the specific nature of the samples used in the two experiments. This replication was undertaken in order to verify the generalizability of the findings of experiment V. It will be recalled that in experiment V, an attitude-toward-French-Canadians scale (FC scale) was used to select a sample of English-Canadian students generally showing a somewhat unfavorable attitude toward French-Canadians. A *directly translated French version* of the same scale, separately standardized on a French-Canadian population (see Dutta *et al.*, 1969), was used in experiment VI to select a sample of French-Canadian students showing highly favorable attitudes toward their own group. It should be noted at this point that in a test of validity of the FC scale, Dutta *et al.* (1969), found that in the case of the English version of the FC scale, the English-Canadian students who had an unfavorable attitude toward French-Canadians also displayed a strong feeling of identification with their own group. Subjects in experiment V were selected from this group. In the case of the French-Canadian subjects, however, a French version of the same FC scale was used and no attempt was made to measure their attitude toward English-Canadians. The validity measure in this case indicated that favorable attitudes of the French-Canadians toward themselves were associated with a strong feeling of identification with their own group. It was noted by the authors, however, that although an unfavorable attitude towards a supposedly rival group may reasonably be considered as involving a strong feeling of identification with one's own group, a favorable attitude towards one's own group does not necessarily have to be accompanied by an unfavorable attitude toward the other. Thus, while there is evidence that the English-Canadian sample of experiment V not only identified with its own group but also had negative attitudes towards French-Canadians, it cannot be assumed that the strong identification of the French-Canadian sample of experiment VI with its own group was accompanied by negative attitudes towards English-Canadians. In any case, the attitude-toward-French-Canadians scale was used in selecting English-Canadians showing unfavorable attitudes towards the French-Canadians in experiment V and French-Canadian students showing favorable attitudes towards their own group in experiment VI. Since our purpose was simply to ensure some degree of emotional involvement on the part of subjects in the experimental situation, the latter group of subjects was considered to be as suitable as the former.

Method

Subjects. On the basis of the French version of the FC scale mentioned above, 120 French-Canadian undergraduate students from the University of

Montreal showing highly favorable attitudes toward their own group were selected from a total of 263 students. A period of 2 months intervened between the administering of the attitude scale on the original group and the experiment conducted on the sample of 120 subjects. The entire study was conducted by one member of the teaching staff and a few graduate students of the Department of Psychology in University of Montreal. None of the people who administered the attitude scale, however, had anything to do with the subsequent experiment. Fifty-two of the subjects were females and 68 males. Their mean age was 18.71 years.

Materials. Materials used in this experiment were the same as in the previous experiment except for the fact that everything was directly translated into French. Most of the adjectives used were translations or close equivalents in French of those used in experiment V.

Procedure and design. Again, the procedure and design followed in experiment VI were the same in every minute detail as used in Experiment V. The only variation was that the experimenter and his confederate were graduate students of the University of Montreal.

The same set of hypotheses as tested in experiment V were considered again in experiment VI. The specific predictions, of course, had to be adjusted in consistency with the nature of the sample used in this experiment as distinguished from that used in the previous one. Thus, in the case of subjects in experiment VI, the pattern of affective intensity as well as of recall of pleasant and unpleasant adjectives as attributed to the two socio-linguistic groups should be in the opposite direction to that observed in the case of subjects in experiment V. Specifically, among the adjectives attributed to FC in the case of GI in experiment IV pleasant adjectives would be perceived as more intensely affective and would also be recalled more frequently by students as compared to unpleasant adjectives; conversely, when attributed to EC, pleasant adjectives would tend to be perceived as having less intense affect and would also be recalled less frequently by them as compared to unpleasant adjectives. Similarly, each of the other predictions in experiment VI should be contrasted with the corresponding prediction in experiment V.

Results

The results of experiment VI are presented in the same manner as in experiment V. Thus each table in this experiment may be directly compared with the corresponding table in the previous one.

Perceived intensity of affect. A three-way analysis of variance was performed on the initial ratings of the adjectives by 24 subjects in each of GI and GII. The results of the analysis presented in Table 34 show that one main effect and two interaction effects were significant. It should be noted that whereas in experiment V the P/U effect (i.e., B) was significant and the EC/FC (i.e., A) was insignificant, in experiment VI the latter was found to be significant and the former was not. The significance of FC/EC in this case was

Table 34. *Analysis of Variance of Initial Ratings of Affective Intensity (GI and GII)*

Sources of variation	Sums of squares	d.f.	MS	*F*
Between S:	60.193	47		
GI/GII (C)	3.510	1	3.510	2.849
Error (b)	56.683	46	1.232	
Within S:	36.565	144		
FC/EC (A)	1.576	1	1.576	6.882*
P/U (B)	0.005	1	0.005	0.029
A × B	9.373	1	9.373	72.659**
A × C	0.020	1	0.020	0.087
B × C	0.490	1	0.490	2.816
A × B × C	0.614	1	0.614	4.760*
Error (w)	24.487	138		
Error 1 (w)	10.544	46	0.299	
Error 2 (w)	8.016	46	0.174	
Error 3 (w)	5.927	46	0.129	
Total	96.758	191		

** $p < 0.01$. * $p < 0.05$.

due to the fact that adjectives (taking P and U together) attributed to FC were perceived, on the whole, by subjects as having greater affective intensity than those attributed to EC. Except for this one shift of significance from one main effect in experiment V to the other in experiment VI, the results of the two analyses were virtually identical. The most crucial and relevant effect from our point of view, i.e., the A × B interaction effect, was found to be significant in this case confirming the same effect observed in experiment V (compare Table 34 with Table 14). The absence of any significant effect of GI/GII (i.e., C) and its interaction with either of the two main experimental variables (i.e., A × C and B × C) is also consistent with the results obtained in experiment V. Finally, in both the experiments the triple interaction was significant. That the reason for this effect is the same as in experiment V will

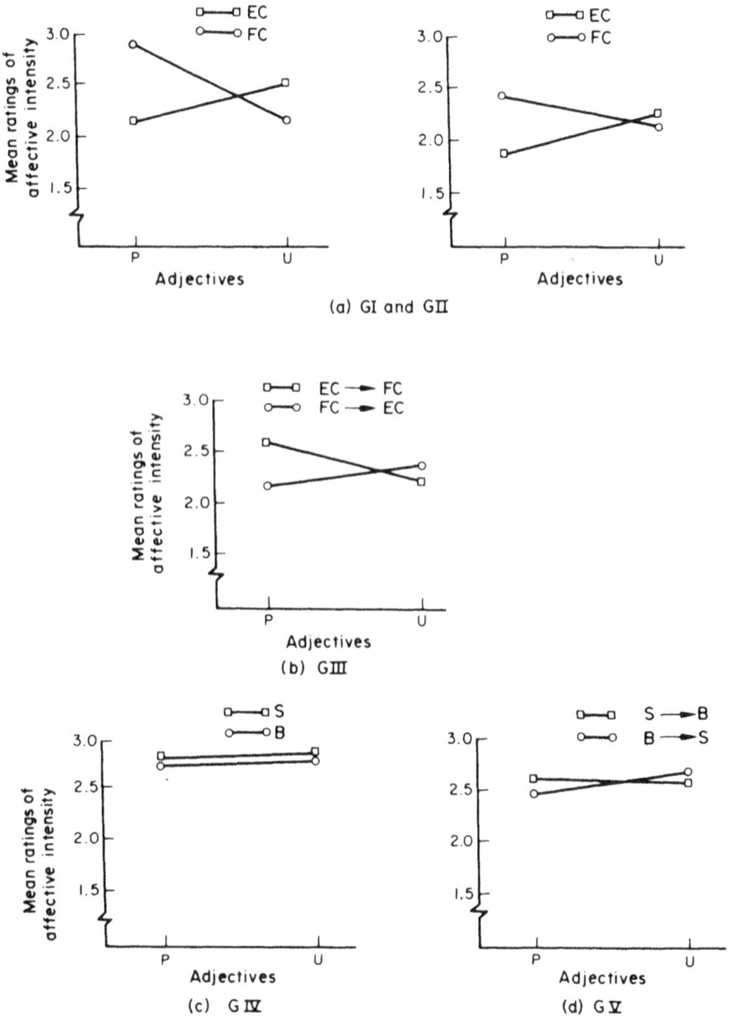

Fig. 4. Affective intensity ratings of P and U adjectives (experiment VI).

become obvious if Fig. 4a, representing the comparisons of average mean intensities of affect, is consulted. The results revealed that each of the predicted differences was significant in both GI and GII; but the magnitude of the difference between the affective intensity of P and that of U adjectives attributed to FC in GII was considerably less than that obtained in the corresponding category in GI, thus resulting in a significant triple interaction effect. Table 35 summarizes the comparisons between the means of the affective intensity of adjectives in different categories for both GI and GII. The results obtained in experiment V regarding the initial ratings of affective intensity were thus replicated in experiment VI (compare Table 15 with Table 35 and Figure 2a with Figure 4a).

Table 35. *Comparisons of Intensity of Affect of Pleasant and Unpleasant Adjectives During Initial Rating Stage (GI and GII)*

Group	Adjectives attributed to		Adjectives P	Adjectives U	*t*
I	FC	M	2.914	−2.247	6.413***
		SD	0.451	0.595	
	EC	M	2.198	−2.641	4.260***
		SD	0.710	0.578	
II	FC	M	2.449	−2.211	2.288*
		SD	0.550	0.698	
	EC	M	1.919	−2.338	4.029***
		SD	0.736	0.895	

*** $p < 0.001$. * $p < 0.05$.

Hypothesis 1, supported in experiment V, is thus confirmed in experiment VI.

The results of a three-way analysis of variance performed on the subsequent ratings of adjectives by GIII are presented in Table 36. It will be observed that one of the main effects, i.e., A, and the interaction effect, i.e., A × B, were found to be significant. The former effect results from the fact that the adjectives (taking P and U together) *originally attributed to EC* and later reported as characterizing FC, were perceived by the Ss, on the whole, as more intensely affective as compared to the adjectives *originally attributed to FC* and later stated to be the characteristics of EC. It may be recalled that in experiment V neither of the main effects was significant (compare Table 36 and Table 16). The significant interaction effect in this case, however, was consistent with the same effect observed in experiment V. Comparisons of the average mean intensities of affect presented graphically in Fig. 4b clearly show that all the differences were in the predicted directions and consistent with the subsequent ratings of GIII in experiment V (compare Fig. 2b and 4b). Table 37 summarizes the results corresponding to Fig. 4b. It will be observed that only one of the differences in the present case was statistically significant. Despite the somewhat unexpected reduction in the magnitudes of the differences, the essential similarity between the two sets of results (compare Table 37 and Table 17) is strongly suggestive with regard to the consistency of results obtained in the two experiments.

Hypothesis 2, verified in experiment V, is thus reinforced by the findings in experiment VI.

Table 36. *Analysis of Variance of Subsequent Ratings of Affective Intensity (GIII)*

Sources of variation	Sums of squares	d.f.	MS	*F*
Between (S)	28.154	23		
Within:	11.634	72		
FC→EC/EC→FC (A)	0.779	1	0.779	4.556*
P/U (B)	0.034	1	0.034	0.362
A × B	1.366	1	1.366	9.356**
A × S	3.941	23	0.171	
B × S	2.151	23	0.094	
A × B × S	3.363	23	0.146	
Total	39.788	95		

** $p < 0.01$. * $p < 0.05$.

Table 37. *Comparisons of Intensity of Affect of Pleasant and Unpleasant Adjectives during Subsequent Rating Stage (GIII)*

Group		Adjectives		*t*
		P	U	
FC → EC	M	2.210	-2.411	1.827
	SD	0.632	0.662	
EC → FC	M	2.629	-2.353	2.509*
	SD	0.608	0.656	

* $p < 0.02$.

Table 38. *Average Mean Intensities of Affect of Pleasant and Unpleasant Adjectives During Initial Rating Stage (GIV)*

Group		Adjectives	
		P	U
S	M	2.834	-2.902
	SD	0.410	0.566
B	M	2.775	-2.878
	SD	0.439	0.528

Table 39. *Average Mean Intensities of Affect of Pleasant and Unpleasant Adjectives During Subsequent Rating Stage (GV)*

Group		Adjectives	
		P	U
S → B	M	2.639	-2.605
	SD	0.560	0.544
B → S	M	2.498	-2.719
	SD	0.516	0.523

The results of a three-way analysis of variance performed on the initial ratings by GIV revealed that, as in experiment V, none of the effects was statistically significant. Similar nonsignificant effects were obtained when an analysis of variance was performed on the subsequent ratings by GV; this, again, was entirely in accordance with what was observed in experiment V.

Average mean intensities of affect initially rated by GIV are presented graphically in Fig. 4c and those subsequently rated by GV are presented in Fig. 4d. Comparisons of the former figure with Fig. 2c and the latter with Fig. 2d will clearly show the essential similarity between the results obtained in the two experiments. Tables 38 and 39 summarize the results corresponding to Fig. 4c and d, respectively. Comparisons between Table 18 and 38 as well as between Tables 19 and 39 would also demonstrate that the results regarding affective intensity ratings of GIV and GV were essentially identical in the two experiments.

Thus, as in the case of experiment V, the initial ratings of GIV and the subsequent ratings of GV in experiment VI together confirm hypothesis 3.

Table 40. *Analysis of Variance of Recall Scores (GI)*

Sources of variation	Sums of squares	d.f.	MS	F
Between (S)	42.958	23		
Within:	80.000	72		
FC/EC (A)	0.166	1	0.166	0.559
P/U (B)	0.375	1	0.375	0.519
A × B	32.667	1	32.667	32.216**
A × S	6.834	23	0.297	
B × S	16.625	23	0.723	
A × B × S	23.333	23	1.014	
Total	122.958	95		

** $p < 0.01$.

Table 41. *Comparisons of Pleasant and Unpleasant Recalls Under Two Different Conditions (GI)*

Group		Adjectives		t
		P	U	
FC	M	2.875	1.583	4.440***
	SD	0.992	1.018	
EC	M	1.792	2.833	3.577***
	SD	1.215	0.638	

*** $p < 0.001$.

Table 42. *Analysis of Variance of Recall Scores (GII)*

Sources of variation	Sums of squares	d.f.	MS	F
Between (S)	39.333	23		
Within:	46.500	72		
FC → EC/EC → FC (A)	0.375	1	0.375	1.201
P/U (B)	0.166	1	0.166	0.208
A × B	7.042	1	7.042	12.038**
A × S	7.125	23	0.310	
B × S	18.334	23	0.797	
A × B × S	13.458	23	0.585	
Total	85.833	95		

** $p < 0.01$.

Table 43. *Analysis of Variance of Recall Scores (GIII)*

Sources of variation	Sums of squares	d.f.	MS	F
Between (S)	42.125	23		
Within:	57.500	72		
FC → EC/EC → FC (A)	0.167	1	0.167	0.312
P/U (B)	0.042	1	0.042	0.102
A × B	20.166	1	20.166	30.234**
A × S	12.333	23	0.536	
B × S	9.458	23	0.411	
A × B × S	15.334	23	0.667	
Total	99.625	95		

** $p < 0.01$.

Table 44. *Comparisons of Pleasant and Unpleasant Recalls Under Two Different Conditions (GII)*

Group		Adjectives P	Adjectives U	t
FC → EC	M	2.167	2.792	2.828**
	SD	0.867	1.020	
EC → FC	M	2.833	2.375	2.072*
	SD	1.008	0.769	

** $p < 0.01$. * $p < 0.05$.

Table 45. *Comparisons of Pleasant and Unpleasant Recalls Under Two Different Conditions (GIII)*

Group		Adjectives P	Adjectives U	t
FC → EC	M	1.542	2.500	4.059**
	SD	1.102	0.885	
EC → FC	M	2.542	1.667	3.708**
	SD	0.930	0.761	

** $p < 0.01$.

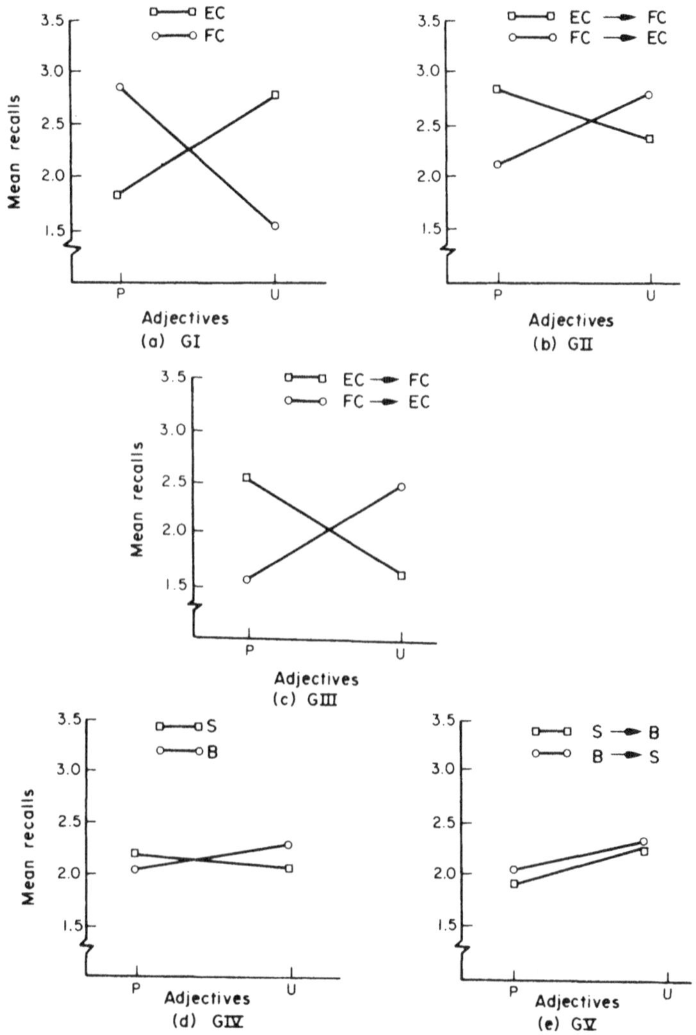

Fig. 5. Selective patterns of recall of P and U adjectives (experiment VI).

Recall. The recall scores for each group in experiment VI were analyzed. The results of a three-way analysis of variance performed on the recall scores of GI have been presented in Table 40. It will be observed that, as in the case of experiment V, only the interaction effect was found to be significant (compare Table 40 with Table 20). The mean recall scores for each of the four categories, calculated over 24 subjects, were presented graphically in Fig. 5a and summarized in Table 34. Each of the predicted differences was found to be statistically significant and the entire pattern of recall was in complete conformity with that obtained in experiment V (compare Table 11 with Table 41 and Fig. 3a with Fig. 5a). The implications of the pattern of recalls, obtained from GI in the present experiment, were the same as stated in detail in the discussion of experiment V.

Hypothesis 4(a) is thus supported by the observed recall pattern of GI exactly as in the case of experiment V.

Separate analyses of variance were performed on the recall scores of GII and GIII and presented in Tables 42 and 43, respectively. In each case, as in experiment V, only the interaction effect was found to be statistically significant (compare Tables 22 and 23 with Tables 42 and 43, respectively). When the mean recall scores under different conditions within each group were compared, as graphically presented in Fig. 5b and c, respectively, it was observed that the patterns of differential recalls for the two groups were essentially the same. The results summarized in Tables 44 and 45 show that, in conformity with the predictions and consistent with the results obtained in experiment V, the differences were significant in both groups. Thus, the recall scores of GII and GIII confirmed the results obtained in experiment V as well as their implications (compare Fig. 5b and c with Fig. 3b and c, and Tables 44 and 45 with Tables 24 and 25, respectively).

The recalls of GII and GIII in experiment VI, therefore, supported hypothesis 4(b) already confirmed in experiment V.

The analysis of the recall scores of GIV and GV, the two groups under low emotional involvement, revealed nonsignificant effects. The nonsignificant effects obtained in each group were again in harmony with the effects obtained in the previous experiment. The mean recalls of GIV and GV presented in Fig. 5d and e (for corresponding tables, consult Tables 46 and 47 respectively) show the uniformity of distribution of the recall scores over different conditions in each case. Thus, in the case of the two groups under low emotional involvement, the patterns of recall obtained in the two experiments were in agreement with each other. Comparisons of Fig. 5d and e with Fig. 3d and e as well as of Tables 46 and 47 with Tables 26 and 27,

Table 46. *Comparisons of Pleasant and Unpleasant Recalls Under Two Different Conditions (GIV)*

		Adjectives	
Group		P	U
S → B	M	2.208	2.125
	SD	1.022	0.947
B → S	M	2.083	2.292
	SD	1.060	0.998

Table 47. *Comparisons of Pleasant and Unpleasant Recalls Under Two Different Conditions (GV)*

		Adjectives	
Group		P	U
S → B	M	1.917	2.292
	SD	0.880	0.623
B → S	M	2.083	2.375
	SD	1.060	1.013

Table 48. *Analysis of Variance of Total Recall Scores (GII, GIII, GIV, and GV)*

Sources of variation	Sums of squares	d.f.	MS	*F*
High versus low emotional involvement (A)	6.511	1	6.511	1.188
Reversal after versus before rating (B)	23.011	1	23.011	4.199*
A × B	21.093	1	21.093	3.849
Error	504.125	92	5.480	
Total	554.740			

* $p < 0.05$.

respectively, will make the similarity between the recall patterns obtained from the same two groups in the two experiments apparent.

Thus, hypothesis 4(c), tested and verified in experiment V, is supported by the results obtained in experiment VI as well.

Total recall. As in the case of experiment V, a two-way analysis of variance was performed on the total recall scores of the four major experimental groups representing the 2 X 2 factorial design (i.e., GII, GIII, GIV, and GV). The results of the analysis presented in Table 48 revealed that the same main effect as in experiment V was significant (compare Table 48 with Table 28). The significance of this effect resulted from the fact that the total recalls of GII and GIV were again found to be greater than those of GIII and GV. The mean recalls of the four groups are presented in Table 49. It will be observed that, as in experiment V, under each of the two levels of emotional involvement, the group that received the reversal information after rating, performed better than the one that received it before rating (compare Table 49 and Table 29). Although in the present case one of the differences was found to be nonsignificant, the overall trend was consistent with that in experiment V. The consistency of this effect in the two experiments emphasizes the necessity of a careful and adequate investigation of the determinants underlying this unexpected phenomenon. Such an investigation, though beyond the scope of the present study, may have significant relevance to the general area of memory organization and reorganization.

Affective intensity and recall. As in the case of experiment V, the most crucial support for the intensity hypothesis as related to retrieval was found here from the test of hypothesis 5. The mean intensities of affect of recalled and nonrecalled adjectives for GI, GIII, and GV are compared in Tables 50, 51, and 52 respectively. In all cases the mean intensities were greater for recalled adjectives than for nonrecalled adjectives. With two exceptions, this was also the same where comparisons were made within categories. If Tables 50, 51, and 52 are compared to Tables 30, 31, and 32, similarity of the results in the two experiments will be apparent.

Thus, hypothesis 5, supported in the previous experiment, found further confirmation in the results obtained in this experiment.

After they had rated the adjectives, GII received reversal information and it was expected that a resulting change in the affective context of the adjectives would eliminate a relationship between the prior rating and retrieval that would otherwise hold. As in the corresponding GII of experiment V, this expectation was fulfilled. The 244 adjectives recalled had a mean affect rating of 2.188 (SD = 0.953); the mean of the 236 adjectives not recalled was 2.272 (SD = 0.910). The difference between these means was not significant ($t = 0.988$, $p > 0.05$).

Group IV also had reversal information subsequent to rating; but in this case the reversal from one affectively neutral context to another was expected to have no effect on the perceived affective intensity of the adjectives. Thus, the relationship between the ratings and recall should be maintained. The mean affective intensity of 209 recalled adjectives was found to be 3.073 (SD = 0.867) which was significantly higher than the mean affective intensity (M = 2.673, SD = 0.869) of the nonrecalled adjectives ($t = 5.000$, $p < 0.001$). The results for GIV thus gave indirect support for the contention that under conditions of low emotional involvement (GIV and GV) the reversal information did not produce any change in the perceived affective intensities of the adjectives. It is to be noted that the results obtained in the previous experiment were confirmed by the above results.

Discussion

It was shown in both experiments that in the context of emotional involvement, interchanging the attributes of the two groups, namely, English-Canadians and French-Canadians, was effective in bringing about changes in the perceived intensities of affect and that retrieval could be directly accounted for by the affective intensities as perceived by subjects at the time of retrieval.

It may be recalled that in the case of groups II and IV, in both the experiments, the reversal information was orally presented to subjects after their last exposure to the adjectives; unlike groups III and V, they were not exposed to the opportunity of acquiring the new information through the process of rating the adjectives subsequent to the reversal information. Thus, the effect of oral information regarding the reversal of the context of the affective items already registered by subjects could be studied directly by analyzing the recall patterns of groups II and IV. In the case of group II, the change in attribution of the adjectives from one emotionally relevant group to another was alone sufficient to reverse the pattern of recall of pleasant and unpleasant adjectives, and to eliminate the relationship found in other groups between the ratings of the affective intensity of the adjectives and their retrieval. In the case of group IV, the attribution of the adjectives was merely changed from one emotionally neutral group to another, and this reversal, presumably having no effect on the perceived intensity of the adjectives, had no effect on either the pattern of recall or the relationship between ratings and recall.

Table 49. *Comparisons of Total Recalls Under Four Treatment Combinations (GII, GIII, GIV, and GV)*

	High emotional involvement				Low emotional involvement		
Group	M	SD	*t*	Group	M	SD	*t*
II. Reversal after rating	10.167	2.614	2.836 **	IV. Reversal after rating	8.708	2.033	0.061
III. Reversal before rating	8.250	2.707		V. Reversal before rating	8.667	1.902	

** $p < 0.01$.

Table 50. *Comparisons of Intensities of Affect of Recalled and Nonrecalled Items (GI)*

		P				U				P + U			
		n	*M*	*SD*	*t*	*n*	*M*	*SD*	*t*	*n*	*M*	*SD*	*t*
FC	Recalled	69	3.150	0.427	4.520	38	−2.834	0.667	5.506	107	3.037	0.555	8.250
	Nonrecalled	51	2.594	0.885	***	82	−1.975	0.834	***	133	2.212	0.906	***
EC	Recalled	43	2.822	0.824	5.897	68	−2.917	0.778	4.262	111	2.880	0.798	7.791
	Nonrecalled	77	1.849	0.879	***	52	−2.282	0.828	***	129	2.023	0.886	***
Total	Recalled	112	3.024	0.632	8.283	106	−2.887	0.745	7.457	218	2.958	0.690	11.187
	Nonrecalled	128	2.146	0.953	***	134	−2.094	0.845	***	262	2.119	0.901	***

*** $p < 0.001$.

Note: n column gives the total number of recalled or nonrecalled items over 20 subjects. Means of combined (P + U) were calculated from the subject's polarity of ratings disregarding algebraic signs.

Table 51. *Comparisons of Intensities of Affect of Recalled and Nonrecalled Items (GIII)*

		P				U				P + U			
		n	*M*	*SD*	*t*	*n*	*M*	*SD*	*t*	*n*	*M*	*SD*	*t*
FC → EC	Recalled	37	2.486	0.727	2.341	60	−2.561	0.723	1.887	97	2.532	0.727	3.254
	Nonrecalled	83	2.088	0.906	*	60	−2.261	0.984		143	2.161	0.943	***
EC → FC	Recalled	61	2.831	0.691	2.810	40	−2.750	0.703	3.612	101	2.799	0.696	4.890
	Nonrecalled	59	2.418	0.892	**	80	−2.154	0.911	***	139	2.266	0.912	***
Total	Recalled	98	2.701	0.723	4.288	100	−2.637	0.720	3.867	198	2.668	0.725	5.759
	Nonrecalled	142	2.225	0.915	***	140	−2.200	0.944	***	282	2.213	0.929	***

*** $p < 0.001$. ** $p < 0.01$. * $p < 0.05$.

Note: *n* column gives the total number of recalled or nonrecalled items over 20 subjects. Means of combined (P + U) were calculated from the subject's polarity of ratings disregarding algebraic signs.

Table 52. *Comparisons of Intensities of Affect of Recalled and Nonrecalled Items (GV)*

		P				U				P + U			
		n	*M*	*SD*	*t*	*n*	*M*	*SD*	*t*	*n*	*M*	*SD*	*t*
S → B	Recalled	46	2.783	1.008	1.827	55	−2.933	0.856	3.712	101	2.865	0.930	3.273
	Nonrecalled	74	2.550	1.064		65	−2.328	0.906	***	139	2.446	1.000	***
B → S	Recalled	50	2.720	0.759	2.122	57	−3.011	0.754	3.634	107	2.875	0.770	4.076
	Nonrecalled	70	2.338	1.090	*	63	−2.455	0.892	***	133	2.394	1.002	***
Total	Recalled	96	2.750	0.888	2.278	112	−2.973	0.806	5.243	208	2.870	0.852	5.161
	Nonrecalled	144	2.447	1.082	*	128	−2.391	0.901	***	272	2.421	1.000	***

*** $p < 0.001$. * < 0.05.

Note: *n* column gives total number of recalled and nonrecalled items over 20 subjects. Means of combined (P + U) were calculated from the subject's polarity of ratings disregarding algebraic signs.

Although the hypothesized effects were consistently confirmed by the results obtained in both experiments, it was felt that it was necessary to probe more closely into the effect of manipulation of affect following registration in order to arrive at conclusions having more generality. That is, instead of having an affective context to start with and then reversing it following registration, one might expose subjects to items in an emotionally neutral context and, following registration, introduce an affective context for the items. The effect of such manipulation of affect interpolated between registration and retrieval on the pattern of recall could then be studied directly on the basis of the predictions derived from the intensity hypothesis.

Experiment VII

The hypotheses tested in this experiment are stated below.

1. At the initial stage, when the adjectives are presented in a neutral context, the affective intensity of the pleasant adjectives will be perceived as equal to that of the unpleasant adjectives.
2. After the introduction of an affective informational context to the adjectives already exposed to the subjects, differential patterns of recall will be obtained from different experimental groups depending upon the specific content of the information. Thus, (a) the group which is given to understand that the adjectives characterize a rival or competitive socio-linguistic group will recall more unpleasant than pleasant adjectives; (b) the group which is informed that the adjectives are attributed to their own socio-linguistic group will recall more pleasant than unpleasant adjectives; (c) the experimental group which is made to understand that the adjectives are ascribed to a neutral and unfamiliar socio-linguistic group will recall the pleasant and the unpleasant adjectives equally well.

Method

Subjects. Forty-five English-Canadian students volunteered to serve as subjects. In this experiment, no attempt was made to select subjects on the basis of their attitudes towards the FC as measured in terms of the FC scale (Dutta *et al.*, 1969). The reason for eliminating such a selection criterion as followed in the previous two experiments was based on the hopeful assumption that it was not essential to select subjects with unfavorable attitudes toward FC. The fact that subjects were EC was considered as sufficient ground for expecting a reasonable level of involvement on their part in the experimental context directly dealing with the English- or French-Canadian characteristics.

At the time of the experiments, all subjects were taking undergraduate courses at Dalhousie University, Halifax, Nova Scotia. Twenty-two of the subjects were males and 23 females. Their mean age was 19.0 years.

Materials. Seven pleasant and seven unpleasant adjectives were selected from the original list of 20 adjectives presented in Table 13. Some of the adjectives were dropped because of their intrinsic incompatibility with the others. That is, since all the adjectives were to be attributed in this experiment to one socio-linguistic group, only one of the two incompatible adjectives, such as intelligent and stupid, could be retained. The final two sets of adjectives, i.e., pleasant and unpleasant, are listed below:

Pleasant	**Unpleasant**
Intelligent	Unreliable
Gentle	Dirty
Lively	Mean
Cheerful	Immoral
Affectionate	Selfish
Warm	Lazy
Independent	Rude

The two sets of adjectives were matched on the basis of the same criteria as used in experiment V.

A rating booklet was prepared in which all the 14 adjectives were to be rated as in the first experiment. In the present case, however, the adjectives were not designated as attributes of any group. In every other respect, the format of the booklet was exactly the same as in experiment V. Thus, each adjective appeared three times to be rated on three bipolar nine-point evaluative scales, namely, pleasant-unpleasant, good-bad, and favorable-unfavorable. Finally, three separate 3 X 5 index cards were prepared. The content of the first index card was as follows:

> BECK, S. H., and GRAHAM, M. L., A study on group characteristics: the typical socio-cultural traits of the French Canadians, *International Bureau of Ethnic Research Bulletin* 5, 17-23 (1966).

In the case of the other two index cards the words "French Canadians" were replaced by "English Canadians" and "Sikkimese".

Procedure and design. Forty-five subjects were randomly assigned to three groups of 15 subjects each. Following their exposure to the adjectives in an emotionally neutral context, each of the three groups was provided with a relevant affective context to the adjectives. There were altogether four different stages of the experiment as given below. All three groups had to go through each of these four stages. Each subject was treated individually.

(a) *Initial rating stage.* During this stage the same rating booklet was presented to all the three groups, I, II, and III. The written introduction that preceded the rating scales in the booklet is given overleaf.

> We are planning to conduct a small-group research in which we shall be using a set of adjectives that characterize different social groups. However, several features of these adjectives have to be controlled and matched before we can use them in our study. We are seeking your help to achieve this aim.
>
> There have been many studies in the area of social attributes or group characteristics which throw light on the typical traits by which different socio-linguistic or cultural groups can be characterized. One of such studies concerning a specific socio-linguistic group has recently been reported by Beck and Graham in *International Bureau of Ethnic Research Bulletin* (1966), the main findings of which will be presented to you. On the basis of extensive investigation, the authors of this study have proposed a set of attributes in terms of which the specific group studied can be characterized. We shall first ask you to rate these adjectives on some evaluative scales without revealing the identity of the socio-linguistic group to which they apply. The name of the group and the complete reference of the study will be revealed to you only after you finish rating the adjectives attributed to the group.

The subjects were given approximately 12 minutes to rate the 14 adjectives over three different evaluative scales included in the booklet. At the end of this initial rating stage, the booklets were collected from subjects.

(b) *Introduction of context.* At this time the name of the socio-linguistic group supposedly characterized by the adjectives rated by subjects was revealed to them. The subjects in group I were provided with the index card attributing the traits to French-Canadians; group II received the card attributing the traits to English-Canadians; and group III received the card attributing the traits to Sikkimese. It was suggested to these subjects that it would be a good idea for them to write down the complete reference of the study since it might be of some relevance to them on some future occasion. Altogether, 5 minutes were devoted to this stage of the experiment, at the end of which the index cards were taken from the subjects.

(c) *Recall.* Each subject in all the three groups was next provided with a recall sheet. The subjects were allowed 5 minutes for free recall of the adjectives attributed to a specific socio-linguistic group and already rated by them. They were not required to follow any order or sequence but merely to write down as many adjectives as they could recall. At the end of the 5-minute period the recall sheet was taken from the subjects.

(d) *Subsequent rating of adjectives.* At this stage, each of the subjects in groups I, II, and III were again provided with the rating booklet, this time without the introduction, and were asked to rate. The subjects were given approximately 12 minutes to finish rating, after which the booklets were collected from them.

It was recognized that the measurement of affective intensity at this stage would be confounded, rendering the results difficult to interpret in unambiguous terms. For instance, any change in affective intensity from the first to the second rating could be attributed to any one or some combination of the following factors: (i) some influence exerted by the subjects' prior ratings of the same adjectives; (ii) the hypothesized effect of the interpolated affective information; and (iii) selective recall of the adjectives by the subjects preceding this rating. Thus, even if the affective intensity ratings at this stage are found to be changed in the predicted directions, one would not be able to argue unequivocally that such ratings reflect the pattern of affective intensity as perceived by the subjects immediately *prior* to their recall of the adjectives. The reason for incorporation of this dubious second rating was not to verify or confirm any of our hypotheses, but merely to extract some additional, incidental, and partial information concerning the data.

As before, the experiment was conducted in an incidental learning context, and care was taken to avoid giving any impression to the subject any time before the recall stage that he would be asked to recall the adjectives later.

Results.

At the initial rating stage, 15 subjects in each of the three experimental groups rated 14 adjectives (seven P and seven U). Thus, each adjective was rated by 45 subjects on three bipolar evaluative scales. As in the previous experiments, each subject's rating score for each adjective was the mean of its intensity ratings over three scales. Each subject had two different mean intensity rating scores (one calculated over seven P adjectives and the other over seven U adjectives). A two-way analysis of variance (Lindquist, 1953; type I design, pp. 267-273) was performed on the initial ratings of the adjectives by the subjects. One of the classifications was three experimental groups and the other was P versus U adjectives. The results revealed that none of the effects was significant.

For each experimental group, the average mean intensity for P as well as for U adjectives was calculated. Comparisons of the two means for each of the three groups are presented separately in Table 53. It will be observed that in none of the groups was the difference between the average mean intensity of the P adjectives and that of U adjectives found to be significant. These results support hypothesis 1.

The recall scores for the three groups were analyzed in the same way. The results of the analysis presented in Table 54 revealed that only the interaction effect was significant. The significant interaction resulted from the fact that the three groups differed from each other with respect to the pattern of

Table 53. *Comparisons of Intensity of Affect of Pleasant and Unpleasant Adjectives During Initial Rating (GI, GII, and GIII)*

Group		Adjectives		t
		P	U	
I	M	2.681	-2.829	1.526
	SD	0.338	0.629	
II	M	2.365	-2.476	1.144
	SD	0.462	0.607	
III	M	2.615	-2.599	0.165
	SD	0.564	0.653	

Table 54. *Analysis of Variance of Recall Scores (GI, GII, and GIII)*

Sources of variation	Sums of squares	d.f.	MS	F
Between S:	58.600	44		
GI/GII/GIII (B)	0.867	2	0.434	0.316
Error (b)	57.733	42	1.374	
Within S:	51.500	45		
P/U (A)	0.011	1	0.011	0.014
A × B	18.155	2	9.078	11.433**
Error (w)	33.334	42	0.794	
Total	110.100	89		

** $p < 0.01$.

relative recalls of P and U adjectives. For each of the three experimental conditions, separate comparisons of P and U mean recalls were made and the results of such comparisons are summarized in Table 55. It will be observed that in the case of GI, where the adjectives were attributed to the FC following the initial rating stage, the subjects recalled U adjectives to a significantly greater extent than P adjectives ($t = 3.692, p < 0.001$). In GII, the adjectives were attributed to EC, and here the subjects recalled more P than U adjectives ($t = 2.871, p < 0.01$). Finally, the subjects in GIII, after being informed that the adjectives were attributed to an Asian community, Sikkimese, recalled P and U adjectives equally well ($t = 1.028, p > 0.05$). Thus, hypotheses 2(a), 2(b), and 2(c) were confirmed by the results.

Table 55. *Comparisons of P and U Recalls Under Three Different Experimental Conditions (GI, GII, and GIII)*

Group		Adjectives		t
		P	U	
		Attributed to FC		
I	M	4.133	5.333	3.692***
	SD	0.917	0.901	
		Attributed to EC		
II	M	5.133	4.200	2.871**
	SD	0.836	1.207	
		Attributed to S		
III	M	5.067	4.733	1.028
	SD	1.162	1.164	

*** $p < 0.001$. ** $p < 0.01$.

Although the initial ratings of none of the three experimental groups showed any difference between the perceived affective intensity of P items and U items, the recall patterns of the three groups following relevant information did differ from each other with respect to differential magnitudes of P and U recalls. On the basis of the intensity hypothesis substantiated by the findings of the first two experiments, one has to infer that differential recall patterns of the three groups resulted from the differences in affective intensity that were brought about in the predicted directions by the relevant affective information following the initial rating stage. For instance, in the case of GI, greater recall of U over P adjectives may be explained by the indirect inference based on the previous findings that the affective intensities of the adjectives underwent changes following the presentation of the informational context. Thus, P adjectives, initially rated to be of equal affective intensity to that of U adjectives, were perceived by subjects to be less intense in affect as compared to the latter subsequent to the introduction of new affective context to the adjectives. Consequently, U adjectives were recalled by them to a greater extent than P adjectives. Similarly, in the case of GII, due to the changes brought about in the affective intensities of adjectives by the relevant information, P adjectives were perceived by the subjects in this group as more intense than U adjectives which led to greater recall of the former as compared to the latter. Finally, in the case of GIII, the informational context was affectively neutral from the standpoint of subjects.

Thus, the perceived intensities of affect of the adjectives as initially rated by subjects did not undergo any changes following their exposure to the new information. Since P and U adjectives were still perceived as equally intense, they were recalled by subjects to the same extent. All these inferences are clearly indirect; and yet, in view of the previous findings indicating a direct relationship between perceived intensity of affect and recall pattern, the inferences seem to be warranted. In fact, the differential recall patterns of the three groups can hardly be explained except in terms of such inferences.

In this connection, the affective intensity ratings for each of the groups during the subsequent rating stage may be considered. Although, as mentioned earlier, this measure may be influenced by the prior ratings or recall, any observed consistency between the predicted and the actual changes in the pattern of affective intensity for each group could certainly be considered as strongly suggestive.

A two-way analysis of variance was performed on the subsequent ratings of the three groups. The results of the analysis presented in Table 56 revealed that the interaction effect was significant. This interaction may be contrasted with the lack of any such effect during the initial rating stage. Comparisons between the average mean intensities of P and those of U adjectives for the three groups, as presented in Table 57, indicate changes in affective intensities in the predicted directions. In the case of GI, the subjects perceived U adjectives as having more intense affect than P adjectives ($t = 2.957$, d.f. = 42. $p < 0.01$). Thus the pattern of affective intensity was entirely consistent with the recall pattern for the group that was informed that the adjectives characterized the FC. In the case of GII, however, although the difference

Table 56. *Analysis of Variance of Subsequent Ratings of Affective Intensity (GI, GII, and GIII)*

Sources of variation	Sums of squares	d.f.	MS	*F*
Between S:	17.144	44		
GI/GII/GIII (B)	1.864	2	0.932	2.560
Error (b)	15.280	42	0.364	
Within S:	10.886	45		
P/U (A)	0.035	1	0.035	0.174
A × B	2.369	2	1.184	5.890**
Error (w)	8.462	42	0.201	
Total	28.030	89		

** $p < 0.01$.

Table 57. *Comparisons of Intensity of Affect of Pleasant and Unpleasant Adjectives During Subsequent Rating (GI, GII, and GII)*

Group		Adjectives P	Adjectives U	*t*
		Attributed to FC		
I	M	2.513	−2.995	2.957**
	SD	0.312	0.640	
		Attributed to EC		
II	M	2.551	−2.264	1.761
	SD	0.477	0.566	
		Attributed to S		
III	M	2.673	−2.596	0.472
		0.536	0.570	

** $p < 0.01$.

was in the predicted direction, the magnitude of the difference failed to reach the acceptable level of significance ($t = 1.761$, d.f. = 42, $p > 0.05$). Finally, the subjects in GIII, after being exposed to the information that the adjectives were ascribed to Sikkimese, did not perceive P and U adjectives as differing in intensity of affect ($t = 0.472, p > 0.05$).

Again, assuming that the effective ratings of subjects following their recall truly reflected the intensities of affect as perceived by them immediately prior to recall, one could compare the mean affective intensity (calculated on the basis of subsequent ratings) of recalled with that of nonrecalled items for each experimental group. The comparisons are summarized in Table 58. It will be observed that in all three groups the recalled items had higher mean ratings than the nonrecalled items.

Table 58. *Comparisons of Subsequently Rated Intensities of Affect of Recalled and Nonrecalled Items (GI, GII, and GIII)*

Group		M	SD	*t*
I	Recalled	2.993	0.843	4.968**
	Nonrecalled	2.362	0.879	
II	Recalled	2.534	0.873	3.123**
	Nonrecalled	2.153	0.735	
III	Recalled	2.787	0.759	4.156**
	Nonrecalled	2.280	0.915	

** $p < 0.01$.

Discussion

Thus, despite an element of ambiguity involved in the measure, the subsequent intensity ratings of subjects in each of the three groups were found to be consistent with the predictions made. The patterns of affective intensity as reflected in the subject's rating at this stage, may be considered, if not as confirmatory, at least as supportive evidence for the phenomenon of change in affective intensity following new affective information.

This experiment was essentially concerned with inquiring into the direct relationship between differential informational exposures following registration of certain items and selective patterns of recall as predicted on the basis of the specific nature of the informational context introduced. The assumption made on the basis of previous findings was that such exposure of subjects to new informational context would bring about changes in the perceived intensities of affect in certain predicted directions and the pattern of recall of each of the experimental groups would be directly determined by such changed patterns of affective intensity. The results showed that although pleasant and unpleasant adjectives were perceived to be of equal affective intensity by each of the groups at the initial stage, their selective recall patterns of pleasant and unpleasant did differ from each other in the predicted directions following exposure to different informational contexts. The predicted changes in the perceived intensities of affect immediately prior to retrieval could not be tested; and yet the subsequent ratings of each of the three experimental groups strongly suggested the occurrence of such changes.

The functional relationship between intensities of affect and retrieval mechanism was the main objective of the inquiry as defined by the three experiments described in this chapter. The results consistently demonstrated that exposure of subjects to new informational context after registration but before retrieval brings about changes in the perceived intensity of affect in certain predicted directions, and the pattern of recall can be directly predicted from such changed patterns of affective intensity. Weiner (1968) has reported some studies on motivated forgetting where changes in informational context introduced following registration did affect the retrieval process. The present investigation went one step further in trying to relate the differential changes in affective intensity of pleasant and unpleasant materials, brought about by different affective contexts introduced before retrieval, to the corresponding patterns of selective recall.

CHAPTER 6

Toward an Integrative Model

A Conceptual Framework

For more than half a century numerous experimental investigations have given rise to diverse theoretical principles regarding the functional relationship between affectivity and memory mechanisms. The failure of most of these studies to make conceptual as well as operational distinctions between different stages of memory has already been noted. Besides, the mutual incompatibility among many of these theoretical positions rendered any accommodation of diverse research findings in this area into a comprehensive as well as consistent explanatory scheme virtually impossible. The intensity hypothesis developed in Chapters 3-5 explains the relationship between emotion and selective memory in terms of perceived intensity of affect, and can be extended to provide a comprehensive framework on the basis of which all the research findings pertinent to the problem could be integrated. Basically, it is proposed that perceived intensity of affect as determined by specific motivational conditions of subjects acts as the immediate antecedent determinant of recall. Whether the variable of task versus ego involvement (Rosenzweig, 1943) as manipulated experimentally, or differential personality dispositions such as strong or weak ego (Alper, 1948) is defined as the independent variable, the consequent affective intensity as an intervening variable can account for the dependent variable of selective recall.

Similarly, whether due to differential frames of reference (Edwards, 1942) or as a result of differential degrees of need achievement (nAch) (Atkinson, 1953), the resultant patterns of affective intensity as differentially perceived by different groups of subjects is suggested as the factor that is directly predictive of their selective patterns of recall. Thus, the intervening variable of perceived intensity of affect can be proposed as the organismic link in terms of which the relationship between diverse independent variables and the dependent variable of recall can be interpreted. A diagrammatical representation of such an integrative conceptual framework is provided in Fig. 6.

In Fig. 6 the interrelationships among the independent, intervening, and dependent variables are summarized. Most of the studies reviewed in the earlier chapters deal with the effects of three kinds of independent variables on selective memory for pleasant and unpleasant materials. One kind of independent variable manipulated in the studies constitutes some form of *organismic predisposition* or relatively more enduring internal state of the individual. The other two kinds of independent variables manipulated in these studies are primarily under the control of the experimenter. One of them can be referred to as a relatively transient motivational state of the individual induced through instructions provided by the experimenter. The third variable refers to the technique used for creating pleasant, unpleasant, or neutral experiences for the individual. Many of the studies, however, have explored the interactive effects of the organismic, the instructional, and the technique variables on selective memory for pleasant and unpleasant materials. But from a purely theoretical point of view, the three sets of variables should be treated independently.

Review of the literature on selective memory suggest three kinds of organismic predisposition variables which have been the focus of attention of researchers. Several studies reviewed in Chapter 2 deal with the role of personality types. Alper (1948), for instance, studied the effects of "strong ego" and "weak ego" on selective retention of pleasant and unpleasant materials. Likewise, Atkinson (1953) has studied the effects of high and low nAch on the recall of pleasant and unpleasant materials. In both the studies of Alper and Atkinson, the authors have paid no attention to the effects of the independent variable on the intervening variable—the perceived intensity of affect. It seems quite reasonable to hypothesize that the kind of effects on selective memory observed in these studies were in fact mediated by the perceived intensity of affect of the materials. Alper (1948) argues that "strong ego" individuals tended to recall more completed (or pleasant) than incompleted (or unpleasant) tasks under ego-orientation and more incompleted than completed tasks under task-orientation, mainly because ego-orientation threatens and task orientation does not threaten the self-esteem of the individual. The reverse pattern however was observed in the case of "weak-ego" individual. The "weak-ego" individual due to his low self-esteem and low frustration tolerance felt threatened by task-orientation and therefore recalled less of incompleted (unpleasant) than completed tasks. Under ego-orientation, the same individual felt too much threatened to avoid the incompleted tasks more than the completed ones. The reasoning can also be applied to hypothesize a similar pattern of results with respect to the intensity of affect of the completed and incompleted tasks. Under ego-orientation, a "strong ego" individual in trying to defend himself, will probably minimize the intensity of affect of an unpleasant experience associated with incompleted tasks, and exaggerate the intensity of affect of a pleasant experience associated with completed tasks. Likewise, he may try to do the reverse under task-orientation. Being faced with a non-threatening situation (under task-orientation), he may take the incompleted tasks more seriously than the completed ones, and therefore may perceive the intensity of affect associated with the former as more intense than the latter. Atkinson's (1953) findings can also be viewed in the same fashion. For instance, Atkinson found that under high achievement conditions, persons with high nAch recalled more incompleted than completed tasks and persons with low nAch recalled more completed than incompleted tasks. This would suggest that a person with low nAch will feel threatened and a person with high nAch will not feel threatened under high achievement conditions. Thus incompletion of a task will be considered as a threat to a low need-achiever and he would therefore act defensively by minimizing the intensity of affect associated with the incompleted task. Similar incompletion of a task, however, will be viewed as a challenge by the high need-achiever. Therefore incompleted tasks may be perceived with more intense affect than completed tasks. These types of postulated relationships between the personality type independent variables and the intervening intensity of affect variable has been suggested in Fig. 6.

A second category of organismic variables refers to relatively enduring social attitudes of the individuals. Several studies (e.g. Edwards, 1941) dealing with the attitudinal variables on selective memory were reviewed in Chapter 2. The experiments discussed in Chapters 4 and 5 revealed the effects of attitudinal variables on both the intensity of affects and recall. Furthermore, the same experiments demonstrated the relationship between the affective intensity of experiences and their selective learning and retrieval.

A third category of organismic variables may be conceptualized in terms of cognitive expectancy of pleasant and unpleasant, or success and failure experiences. Although no study dealing with the effects of cognitive expectancy variables on selective memory has been reported as yet, it is quite reasonable to assume that selective memory for pleasant and unpleasant experiences can be a function of an individual's cognitive expectancies. For example, it seems plausible to hypothesize that from among a set of success and failure experiences, the recallability of success will be low compared to the failures if the individual experienced them under high expectancy of

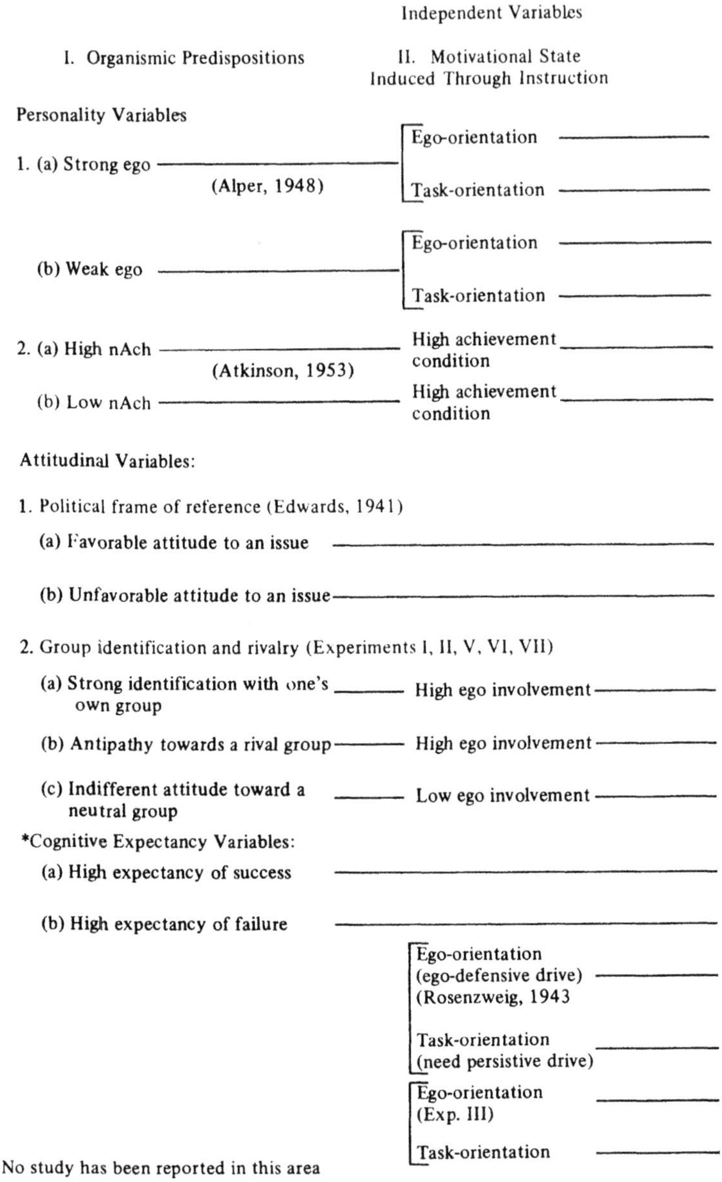

*No study has been reported in this area

Fig. 6. A comprehensive theoretical scheme for

III. Memory Items	Intervening Variable: Perceived Intensity of Affect		Dependent Variable: Selective Recall
__ Completed (or P) tasks / Incompleted (or U) tasks	P > U	(postulated)	P > U
__ Completed (or P) tasks / Incompleted (or U) tasks	U > P		U > P
__ Completed (or P) tasks / Incompleted (or U) tasks	U > P	(postulated)	U > P
__ Completed (or P) tasks / Incompleted (or U) tasks	P > U		P > U
__ Completed (or P) tasks / Incompleted (or U) tasks	U > P	(postulated)	U > P
__ Completed (or P) tasks / Incompleted (or U) tasks	P > U		P > U
__ Favorable (or P) statements / Unfavorable (or U) statements	P > U	(postulated)	P > U
__ Favorable (or P) statements / Unfavorable (or U) statements	U > P		U > P
__ P and U items attributed to self	P > U		P > U
__ P and U items attributed to a rival	U > P	(demonstrated)	U > P
__ P and U items attributed to a neutral group	P > U		P > U
__ Success (or P) tasks / Failure (or U) tasks	U > P	(postulated)	U > P
__ Success (or P) tasks / Failure (or U) tasks	P > U		P > U
__ Completed (or P) tasks / Incompleted (or U) tasks	P > U	(postulated)	P > U
__ Completed (or P) tasks / Incompleted (or U) tasks	U > P		U > P
__ Success (or P) tasks / Failure (or U) tasks	P > U	(demonstrated)	P > U
__ Success (or P) tasks / Failure (or U) tasks	U > P		U > P

retention and retrieval as a function of affective intensity.

success. The reverse, however, will be true under conditions of high expectancy of failure. In other words, on a given task, if the individual expected success but experienced failure, the failure experience would create a stronger impression on him than if he expected to fail in the first place. Likewise, if the individual expected failure but experienced success, the success experience would create a more lasting impression in him than if he expected success before engaging in the task. Thus disconfirmation of an expectancy would create the perception of stronger affect and hence would influence selective memory. The reason why an individual under high expectancy of success would feel failures more intensely and recall them better than successes may lie in the notion of adaptation level (Helson, 1964) of the individual. An individual expects success because of his previous experiences of continuing success. The more success he had in the past, the greater will be his expectation of success, and the less unusual he will feel (or more normal or average he will consider his feelings to be) about his future success. But under these conditions if he fails, he would experience a contrast effect (Sherif and Hovland, 1961), and would consider his failure experience as very unusual and intensely unpleasant.

The development of an expectancy for success and failure or pleasant and unpleasant outcomes associated with experiences is largely determined by an individual's past history of reinforcements. If an individual's life is a series of success stories, he would probably be working most of the time under high expectancy of success. Thus other things being equal, he will probably perceive more intense affect in his failure experiences than in his success experiences, and will recall the former better than the latter. This kind of person is very similar to high need-achiever who is known to have success orientation. On the other hand, an individual, due to his consistent failures in the past may develop a high expectancy of failure (low need-achiever) and may therefore behave exactly in the reverse fashion.

Although cognitive expectancy variable has some parallel in nAch variable, the two should not be equated. Cognitive expectancy for success and failure can be a more transient state in the individual than nAch variable. Besides, cognitive expectancy for success and failure can be manipulated experimentally by controlling the history of reinforcements administered to the individual for his performance on tasks and the effects of such experimentally induced expectancies on intensity of affect and recall of pleasant and unpleasant experiences can then be studied.

The three categories of organismic variables—personality characteristics, social attitudes, and cognitive expectancies—tend to vary on two dimensions.

Firstly, the variables differ with respect to their transient character. Thus personality characteristics are considered as more stable predispositions than attitudes and attitudes are considered as relatively more stable than cognitive expectations of pleasant and unpleasant experiences. Secondly, the variables differ with respect to the ease with which they can be measured and manipulated. The personality variables are the most difficult to pin down and measure in their pure forms. Thus, conceptually one may argue for some pattern of relationship between a personality characteristic and perceived intensity of affect or recall of experiences. But it may become very difficult to empirically verify the relationship due to the difficulties in obtaining an adequate measure of the independent variable. For instance, it is difficult to conclude from the results of experiment IV reported in Chapter 4, that introversion-extroversion dimension is not related to perceived intensity of affect of experiences and their selective recall. In trying to defend Eriksen's (1954) position, one might argue that the measure of the personality variable used in the experiment did not truly reflect the variable that Eriksen had in mind. What is emphasized here is that the studies dealing with the effects of personality variables on selective memory may encounter serious methodological as well as conceptual problems with respect to clarity and precise measurement of the variables. These problems are substantially reduced when one deals with social attitudes and cognitive expectancy variables.

Besides the organismic variables, the studies in the area of selective memory have also used two other kinds of independent variable—instructions provided by the experimenter to create different degrees of involvement for the individual, and different techniques used to create pleasant, unpleasant, or neutral experiences that serve as memory items. These variables tend to interact with organismic disposition variables in producing their effects on both perceived intensity of affect and recall of experiences. These interaction effects are listed in Fig. 6.

Concluding Remarks and Implications

The main concern of the book has been a systematic reformulation of affect-memory relationship. It has been emphasized that this relationship is mediated by the intervening variable of perceived intensity of affect. Assuming that the selective memory process includes three distinct phases of registration, storage, and retrieval, the experiments discussed in Chapters 4 and 5 clearly revealed the effects of intensity of perceived affect on two of the three phases. They demonstrated that the perceived intensity affect not only determined selective learning of experiences, but also determined their retrieval. The procedures utilized in the experiments described in Chapter 5 do not distinguish retrieval effects from storage effects. In fact, until the present time, despite the conceptual distinction between storage and retrieval, it has been considered extremely difficult to distinguish between the two phases in memory in operational terms. Therefore any final statement regarding the generality of the perceived intensity of affect hypothesis as it affects storage phase of the memory as distinguished from retrieval phase, has to be postponed until studies specifically concerned with distinguishing storage and retrieval are conducted.

Further, the theoretical relevance of the implications of the perceived intensity of affect hypothesis to such a concept as arousal, deserves to be explored. It can be speculated at this point that ultimately the physiological correlates of arousal may provide a better and more tangible measure of affective intensity than rating scales. Whether perceived intensity of affect facilitates memory as an autonomic process to be understood in terms of "reverberations" (Hebb, 1949) or such other neural mechanisms or simply as an associative cue made use of by subjects, is also a question to which future studies may fruitfully address themselves. In view of the observed fact in the experiments discussed in Chapter 5 that differential affective intensities as perceived subsequent to item registration by individuals resulted in retrieval patterns entirely consistent with the patterns of affective intensity, the latter explanation, at this point, seems to be more likely. That is, insofar as retrieval has been found to be directly influenced by the perceived pattern of affective intensity introduced following registration, affective intensity may reasonably be conceived to have some cue function that facilitates accessibility or retrieval.

The perceived intensity of affect hypothesis may have implications for such areas as persuasive communication and attitude change. It has been suggested by some investigators (e.g. Janis and Feshback, 1953; Leventhal and Singer, 1966), though not conclusively, that there is a positive relationship between strong affect and the effectiveness of a communication. If affective intensity is considered as the crucial determinant of selective learning and retrieval of information, as suggested in Chapters 4 and 5, then the effectiveness of a message in terms of its being accessible to the receiver may be facilitated by manipulating the degree of affect associated with a message rather than its specific affective quality.

Furthermore, the relevance of the intensity hypothesis to the role of stereotypes in racial prejudice would appear to be obvious on intuitive grounds. Studies by Katz and Braly (1933) and Gilbert (1951) on verbal stereotypes and racial prejudice indicated a strong relationship between the magnitude of undesirability, as perceived by an individual, of the traits or stereotypes attributed to various ethnic groups and the strength of his prejudice against them. Since prejudice is a *learned* response tendency, the stubbornness and persistence of racial prejudice as observed in the reality of our everyday life may perhaps be partially accounted for by the affective intensity of stereotypes that embody such prejudices.

Admittedly, the implications of the intensity hypothesis for a few specific areas of inquiry as suggested above are more speculative than definitive. They are mentioned merely as instances of different lines of exploration related to general problems of social learning and perception. Further investigation of these problems may be benefited by testing the applicability of the perceived intensity of affect hypothesis.

References

Abel, T. M. Neuro-circulatory reaction and the recall of unfinished and completed tasks. *Journal of Psychology* **6**, 377-383 (1938).

Aborn, M. The influence of experimentally induced failure on the retention of material acquired through set and incidental learning. *Journal of Experimental Psychology* **45**, 225-231 (1953).

Alper, T. G. Memory for completed and incompleted tasks as a function of personality: an analysis of group data. *Journal of Abnormal and Social Psychology* **41**, 320-403 (1946a).

Alper, T. G. Task-orientation vs. ego-orientation in learning and retention. *American Journal of Psychology* **59**, 236-248 (1946b).

Alper, T. G. Memory for completed and incompleted tasks as a function of personality: correlation between experimental and personality data. *Journal of Personality* **17**, 104-137 (1948).

Alper, T. G. The interrupted task method in studies of selective recall: a reevaluation of some recent experiments. *Psychological Review* **59**, 71-88 (1952).

Alper, T. G. Predicting the direction of selective recall, its relation to ego strength and N achievement. *Journal of Abnormal and Social Psychology* **55**, 149-165 (1957).

Alper, T. G., and Korchin, S. S. Memory for socially relevant material. *Journal of Abnormal and Social Psychology* **47**, 25-38 (1952).

Amster, H. Evaluative judgment and recall in incidental learning. *Journal of Verbal Learning and Verbal Behavior* **3**, 466-473 (1964).

Atkinson, J. W. The achievement motive and recall of interrupted and completed tasks. *Journal of Experimental Psychology* **46**, 381-390 (1953).

Atkinson, J. W., and Raphelson, A. C. Individual differences in motivation and behavior in particular situations. *Journal of Personality*, 381-390 (1956).

Baddeley, A. D. A Zeigarnik-like effect in the recall of anagram solutions. *Quarterly Journal of Experimental Psychology* **15**, 63-64 (1963).

Bain, A. *The Senses and the Intellect*, Longmans, London, 1868.

Balken, E. R. Affective, volitional and galvanic factors in learning. *Journal of Experimental Psychology* **16**, 115-128 (1933).

Barlow, J. A. Recall of experiences as a function of intensity as compared to quality (pleasantness or unpleasantness) of feeling tone. *Journal of the Scientific Laboratories*, **43**, Arts. 9-12 (Denison University, 1955).

Barnes, J. M., and Underwood, B. J. "Fate" of first-list associations in transfer theory. *Journal of Experimental Psychology* **58**, 97-105 (1959).

Barrett, D. M. Memory in relation to hedonic tone. *Archives of Psychology, New York* **31**, No. 223 (1938).

Bartlett, F. C. *Remembering: A Study in Experimental and Social Psychology*, Cambridge Univ. Press, Cambridge, 1932.

Beebe-Centre, J. G. *The Psychology of Pleasantness and Unpleasantness*, van Nostrand, New York, 1932.

Belmont, L., and Birch, H. G. Reindividualizing the repression hypothesis. *Journal of Abnormal and Social Psychology* **46**, 226-235 (1951).

Bogulavsky, G. W., and Guthrie, E. R. The recall of completed and interrupted activities: an investigation of Ziegarnik's experiment. *Psychological Bulletin* **38**, 575-576 (Abstract) (1941).

Briggs, C. E. Acquisition, extinction, and recovery functions in retroactive inhibition. *Journal of Experimental Psychology* **47**, 418-422 (1954).

Brown, D. R., and Yandell, R. J. Individual perceptual styles following induced failure. *Journal of Personality and Social Psychology* **3**, 359-362 (1966).

Brown, J. Some tests of decay theory of immediate memory. *Quarterly Journal of Experimental Psychology* **10**, 12-21 (1958).

Brown, W. P. Conceptions of perceptual defence. *British Journal of Psychology*, Monograph Supplement, 1961.

Bruner, J. S., and Postman, L. An approach to social perception. In W. Dennis (ed.), *Current Trends in Social Psychology*, University of Pittsburgh Press, Pittsburgh, 1949, pp. 70-119.

Butterfield, E. C. The interruption of tasks: methodological, factual, and theoretical issues. *Psychological Bulletin* **62**, 309-322 (1964).

Cameron, D. E. Remembering. *Nervous and Mental Disease Monograph* **72** (whole No. 22) (1947).

Caron, A. J., and Wallach, M. A. Recall of interrupted tasks under stress: A phenomenon of memory or learning? *Journal of Abnormal and Social Psychology* **55**, 372-381 (1959).

Carter, H. D., and Jones, H. E. A further study of affective factors in learning. *Journal of Genetic Psychology* **50**, 157-163 (1937).

Cartwright, D. The effect of interruption, completion and failure upon the attractiveness of activities. *Journal of Experimental Psychology* **31**, 1-16 (1942).

Cason, H. The learning and retention of pleasant and unpleasant activities. *Archives of Psychology, New York* **21**, No. 134 (1932).

Cason, H., and Lungren, F. C. Memory for pleasant, unpleasant, and indifferent words. *Journal of Experimental Psychology* **15**, 728-732 (1932).

Chaney, R. M., and Lauer, A. R. The influence of affective tone on learning and retention. *Journal of Educational Psychology* **20**, 287-290 (1929).

Dodwell, P. C. Some factors affecting the hearing of words presented dichotically. *Canadian Journal of Psychology* **18**, 72-91 (1964).

Dudycha, G. J., and Dudycha, M. M. Childhood memories: a review of literature. *Psychological Bulletin* **38**, 668-682 (1941).

Dutta, S., and Kanungo, R. N. Retention of affective material: a further verification of the intensity hypothesis. *Journal of Personality and Social Psychology* **5**, 476-481 (1967).

Dutta, S., Norman, L., and Kanungo, R. N. A scale for the measurement of attitudes toward French Canadians. *Canadian Journal of Behavioral Science* **1**, 156-166 (1969).

Dutta, S., Kanungo, R. N., and Freibergs, V. Retention of affective material: effects of intensity on retrieval. *Journal of Personality and Social Psychology* (in press) (1972).

D'Zurilla, T. Recall efficiency and mediating cognitive events in "experimental repression". *Journal of Personality and Social Psychology* **3**, 253-256 (1965).

Edwards, A. L. Political frame of reference as a factor influencing recognition. *Journal of Abnormal and Social Psychology* **36**, 34-50 (1941).

Edwards, A. L. The retention of affective experiences: a criticism and restatement of the problem. *Psychological Review* **49**, 43–53 (1942).

Eriksen, C. W. Psychological defenses and "ego-strength" in the recall of completed and incompleted tasks. *Journal of Abnormal and Social Psychology* **49**, 45-50 (1954).
Eysenck, H. J. *Dimensions of personality.* Routledge & Kegan Paul, London, 1947.
Feather, N. T. Attitude and selective recall. *Journal of Personality and Social Psychology* **12**, 310-319 (1969).
Festinger, L. *A Theory of Cognitive Dissonance*, Stanford University Press, California, 1963.
Flavell, J. Repression and the "return of the repressed". *Journal of Consulting Psychology* **19**, 441-443 (1955).
Fox, C. The influence of subjective preference on memory. *British Journal of Psychology* **13**, 398-404 (1923).
Frank, J. D. Affective value vs. nature of odors in relation to reproduction. *American Journal of Psychology* **43**, 479-483 (1931).
Frank, J. D., and Ludwigh, E. J. The retroactive effect of pleasant and unpleasant odors on learning. *American Journal of Psychology* **43**, 102-108 (1931).
Franks, C. M. Conditioning and abnormal behavior. In H. J. Eysenck (ed.), *Handbook of Abnormal Psychology*, Basic Books, New York, 1961, pp. 457-487.
Freud, S. *On the Psychopathology of Everyday Life*, Macmillan, New York, 1914.
Freud, S. Repression. *In Collected Papers*, Hogarth Press, London, 1925, vol. 4, pp. 84-97.
Gilbert, G. M. The new status of experimental studies on the relationship of feeling to memory. *Psychological Bulletin* **35**, 26-35 (1938).
Gilbert, G. M. Stereotype persistence and change among college students. *Journal of Abnormal and Social Psychology* **46**, 245-254 (1951).
Glickman, S. E. Perseverative neural processes and consolidation of the memory trace. *Psychological Bulletin* **58**, 218-233 (1961).
Glixman, A. F. Recall of completed and incompleted activities under varying degrees of stress. *Journal of Experimental Psychology* **39**, 281-295 (1949).
Goldin, P. C. Experimental investigation of selective memory and the concept of repression and defense. *Journal of Abnormal and Social Psychology* **69**, 365-391 (1964).
Green, D. R. Volunteering and the recall of interrupted tasks. *Journal of Abnormal and Social Psychology* **66**, 392-401 (1963).
Harden, L. M. The effect of emotional reactions upon retention. *Journal of Genetic Psychology* **3**, 197-221 (1930).
Harrower, M. R. Organization in higher mental processes. *Psychologische Forschung* **17**, 56-120 (1932).
Hebb, D. P. *The Organization of Behavior*, Wiley, New York, 1949.
Heider, F. *The Psychology of Interpersonal Relations*, Wiley, New York, 1958.
Helson, H. Current trends and issues in adaptation-level theory. *American Psychologist* **19**, 26-38 (1964).
Henderson, E. N. Do we forget the disagreeable? *Journal of Philosophy, Psychology and Scientific Methods* **8**, 432-437 (1911).
Heyer, A. W., Jr., and O'Kelley, L. T. Studies in motivation and retention: II. Retention of nonsense syllables learned under different degrees of motivation. *Journal of Psychology* **27**, 143-152 (1949).
Hunter, I. M. L. The solving of five-letter anagram problems. *British Journal of Psychology* **50**, 193-206 (1959).
Holmes, D. S. Differential change in effective intensity and the forgetting of unpleasant personal experiences. *Journal of Personality and Social Psychology* **15**, 234-239 (1970).
Holmes, D. S. Repression or interference? A further investigation. *Journal of Personality*

and Social Psychology **22,** 163-170 (1972).

Holmes, D. S., and Schallow, J. Reduced recall after ego-threat: Repression or Response competition? *Journal of Personality and Social Psychology* **13,** 145-152 (1969).

Inglis, J. Abnormalities of motivation and "ego-functions". In H. J. Eysenck (ed.), *Handbook of Abnormal Psychology,* Pittman, London, 1960.

Janis, I. L., and Feshback, S. Effects of fear arousing communications. *Journal of Abnormal and Social Psychology* **48,** 78-92 (1953).

Jersild, A. Memory for the pleasant as compared with the unpleasant. *Journal of Experimental Psychology* **14,** 284-288 (1931).

Jones, E. E., and Aneshansel, J. The learning and utilization of contravaluant material. *Journal of Abnormal and Social Psychology* **53,** 27-34 (1956).

Jourard, S. M. Ego strength and the recall of tasks. *Journal of Abnormal and Social Psychology* **49,** 51-58 (1954).

Kanungo, R. N. Retention of affective material: role of extraversion and intensity of affect. *Journal of Personality and Social Psychology* **8,** 63-68 (1968).

Kanungo, R. N., and Das, J. P. Differential learning and forgetting as a function of the social frame of reference. *Journal of Abnormal and Social Psychology* **61,** 82-86 (1960).

Kanungo, R. N., and Dutta, S. Retention of affective material: frame of reference or intensity? *Journal of Personality and Social Psychology* **4,** 27-35 (1966).

Katz, D., and Braly, K. W. Racial prejudice and racial stereotypes. *Journal of Abnormal and Social Psychology* **30,** 175-193 (1933).

Klugman, S. F. Retention of affectively toned verbal material by normals and neurotics. *Journal of Abnormal and Social Psychology* **53,** 321-327 (1956).

Koch, H. L. The influence of some affective factors upon recall. *Journal of General Psychology* **4,** 171-190 (1930).

Koffka, K. *Principles of Gestalt Psychology,* Harcourt, Brace, New York, 1935.

Leventhal, H., and Singer, R. P. Affect arousal and positioning of recommendations in persuasive communication. *Journal of Personality and Social Psychology* **4,** 137-146 (1966).

Levine, J. M., and Murphy, G. The learning and forgetting of controversial material. *Journal of Abnormal and Social Psychology* **38,** 507-517 (1943).

Lewin, K. *A Dynamic Theory of Personality,* McGraw-Hill, New York, 1935.

Lewis, H. B. An experimental study of the role of the ego in work: I. The role of the ego in cooperative work. *Journal of Experimental Psychology* **34,** 11-26 (1944).

Lewis, H. B., and Franklin, M. An experiment study of the role of the ego in work: II. The significance of task-orientation in work. *Journal of Experimental Psychology* **34,** 195-215 (1944).

Lindquist, E. F. *Design and Analysis of Experiments in Psychology and Education,* Houghton Mifflin, Boston, 1953.

Madison, P. *Freud's Concept of Repression and Defense, Its Theoretical and Observation Language,* University of Minnesota Press, Minneapolis, 1961.

Mandler, G. The interruption of behavior. In M. R. Jones (ed.) *Nebraska Symposium on Motivation,* University of Nebraska Press, Lincole, 1964.

Marrow, A. J. Goal tensions and recall: I. *Journal of General Psychology* **19,** 3-35 (1938a).

Marrow, A. J. Goal tensions and recall: II. *Journal of General Psychology* **19,** 37-64 (1938b).

McClelland, D. C. *Personality,* Sloane, New York, 1951.

McGeoch, J. A. Forgetting and the law of disuse. *Psychological Review* **39,** 352-370 (1932).

McGeoch, J. A., and Irion, A. L. *The Psychology of Human Learning,* Longmans, New York, 1952.
McGranahan, D. V. A critical and experimental study on repression. *Journal of Abnormal and Social Psychology* **35**, 212-225 (1940).
Melton, A. W. Implications of short term memory for a general theory of memory. *Journal of Verbal Learning and Verbal Behavior* **2**, 1-21 (1963).
Melton, A. W., and Irwin, J. McQ. The influence of degree of interpolated learning and retroactive inhibition and the overt transfer of specific responses. *American Journal of Psychology* **53**, 173-203 (1940).
Meltzer, H. The present status of experimental studies on the relationship of feeling to memory. *Psychological Review* **53**, 173-203 (1930).
Menzies, R. N. Memory for pleasant, unpleasant, and indifferent events of the recent past. *Psychological Bulletin* **30**, 574 (1933).
Menzies, R. N. The comparative memory values of pleasant, unpleasant and indifferent experiences. *Journal of Experimental Psychology* **18**, 267-279 (1935).
Merrill, R. M. The effect of pre-experimental and experimental anxiety on recall efficiency. *Journal of Experimental Psychology* **48**, 167-172 (1954).
Moore, E. H. A note on the recall of the pleasant vs. the unpleasant. *Psychological Review* **42**, 214-215 (1935).
Müller, G. E., and Pilzecker, A. Experimentelle Beitrage zur Lehre vom Gedachtnis. *Zeitschrift für Psychologie* **1**, 1-300 (1900).
Nowlis, H. H. The influence of success and failure on the resumption of an interrupted task. *Journal of Experimental Psychology* **28**, 304-325 (1941).
O'Kelley, L. T., and Steckle, L. C. The forgetting of pleasant and unpleasant experiences. *American Journal of Psychology* **53**, 432-434 (1940).
Osgood, C. E. *Method and Theory in Experimental Psychology,* Oxford University Press, New York, 1953.
Osgood, C. E., and Tannenbaum, P. H. The principle of congruity in the prediction of attitude change. *Psychological Review* **62**, 42-55 (1955).
Osgood, C. E., Suci, G. J., and Tannenbaum, P. H. *The Measurement of Meaning,* Univ. of Illinois Press, Urbana, 1957.
Pachauri, A. R. A study of Gestalt problems in completed and interrupted tasks. *British Journal of Psychology* **25**, 365-381, 447-457 (1935).
Pachauri, A. R. A study of Gestalt problems in completed and interrupted tasks: Part III, *British Journal of Psychology* **27**, 170-180 (1936).
Penn, N. Experimental improvements on an analogue of repression paradigm. *Psychological Record* **14**, 185-196 (1964).
Postman, L. The present status of interference theory. In C. N. Cofer (ed.), *Verbal Learning and Verbal Behavior,* McGraw-Hill, New York, 1961, pp. 152-179.
Prentice, W. C. H. Retroactive inhibition and the motivation of learning. *American Journal of Psychology* **56**, 283-292 (1943).
Rapaport, D. *Emotion and Memory,* International Univ. Press, New York, 1959.
Ratliff, M. M. The varying function of affectively toned olfactory, visual and auditory cues in recall. *American Journal of Psychology* **51**, 695-701 (1938).
Rosenthal, B. G. Hypnotic recall of material learned under anxiety and non-anxiety producing conditions. *Journal of Experimental Psychology* **33**, 369-389 (1944).
Rosenzweig, S. Preference in repetition of successful and unsuccessful activities as a function of age and personality. *Journal of Genetic Psychology* **42**, 421-441 (1933a).
Rosenzweig, S. The recall of finished and unfinished tasks as affected by the purpose with which they were performed. *Psychological Bulletin* **30**, 698 (1933b).
Rosenzweig, S. The preferential repetition of successful and unsuccessful activities.

Psychological Bulletin **33,** 797 (1936).

Rosenzweig, S. The experimental study of repression. In *Explorations in Personality*, Oxford Univ. Press, New York, 1938.

Rosenzweig, S. Need-persistive and ego-defensive reactions to frustration as demonstrated by an experiment in repression. *Psychological Review* **48,** 347-349 (1941).

Rosenzweig, S. An experimental study of "repression" with special reference to need-persistive and ego-defensive reactions to frustration. *Journal of Experimental Psychology* **32,** 64-74 (1943).

Rosenzweig, S., and Mason, G. A. An experimental study of memory in relation to the theory of repression. *British Journal of Psychology* **24,** 247-265 (1934).

Sears, R. R. Functional abnormalities of memory with special reference to amnesia. *Psychological Bulletin* **33,** 229-274 (1936).

Sherif, M., and Hovland, C. I. *Social Judgment: Assimilation and Contrast Effects in Communication and Attitude Change,* Yale University Press, New Haven, 1961.

Silverman, A., and Cason, H. Incidental memory for pleasant, unpleasant and indifferent words. *American Journal of Psychology* **46,** 315-320 (1934).

Spencer, H. *The Principles of Psychology,* Appleton, New York, 1873.

Stagner, R. The redintegration of pleasant and unpleasant experiences. *American Journal of Psychology* **43,** 463-468 (1931).

Stone, A. R. The reaction of memory to affective states. *American Journal of Psychology* **36,** 112-123 (1925).

Taft, R. Selective recall and memory distortion of favorable materials. *Journal of Abnormal and Social Psychology* **49,** 23-28 (1954).

Thomson, R. H. An experimental study of memory as influenced by feeling tone. *Journal of Experimental Psychology* **13,** 462-468 (1930).

Thorndike, E. L. *Educational Psychology,* Vol. I: *The Original Nature of Man,* Teach. Coll. Press, New York, 1923.

Thorndike, E. L. The law of effect. *American Journal of Psychology,* **39,** 212-222 (1927).

Thorndike, E. L., and Lorge, I, *The Teacher's Wordbook of 30,000 Words,* Teacher's College, Columbia University, New York, 1944.

Truax, C. B. The repression response to implied failure as a function of the hysteria-psychasthenia index. *Journal of Abnormal and Social Psychology* **55,** 188-193 (1957).

Turner, R. H., and Barlow, J. H. Memory for pleasant and unpleasant experiences: some methodological considerations. *Journal of Experimental Psychology* **42,** 189-196 (1951).

Underwood, B. J. Interference and forgetting. *Psychological Review* **64,** 49-60 (1957).

Walker, E. L. Action decrement and its relation to learning. *Psychological Review,* **65,** 129-142 (1958).

Washburn, K. F., Giang, F., Ives, M., and Pollock, M. Memory revival of emotions as a test of emotional and phlegmatic temperaments. *American Journal of Psychology* **36,** 454-456 (1925a).

Washburn, M. F., Harding, L., Simmons, H., and Tomlinson, D. Further experiments on directed recall as a test of cheerful and depressed temperaments. *American Journal of Psychology* **36,** 454-456 (1925b).

Waters, R. H., and Leeper, R. The relation of affective tone to the retention of experiences of daily life. *Journal of Experimental Psychology* **19,** 203-215.

Weiner, B., Effects of motivation on the availability and retrieval of memory traces. *Psychological Bulletin* **65,** 24-37 (1966a).

Weiner, B. Motivation and memory. *Psychological Monographs (General and Applied)* **80,** No. 18 (1966b).

Weiner, B. Motivated forgetting and the study of repression. *Journal of Personality* **36,** 213-234 (1968).

White, M. M., and Powell, M. Differential reaction time for pleasant and unpleasant words. *American Journal of Psychology* **48,** 126-133 (1936).

White, M. M., and Ratliff, M. M. The relation of affective tone to the learning and recall of words. *American Journal of Psychology* **46,** 92-98 (1934).

Windgard, E. Recognition memory and recall as a function of degree of polarization on the semantic differential. *Journal of Verbal Learning and Verbal Behavior* **5,** 566-571 (1966).

Wohlgemuth, A. The influence of feeling on memory. *British Journal of Psychology* **2,** 263-271 (1923).

Yamaguchi, H. Completion-incompletion of tasks and pleasant-unpleasant toned feeling in selective recall (summary). *Psychological Reports* **16,** 710 (1965).

Zajonc, R. B. Attitudinal effects of mere exposure. *Journal of Personality and Social Psychology* **8,** monograph, 1-29 (1968).

Zeigarnik, B. On finished and unfinished tasks. In W. D. Ellis (ed.), *A Source Book of Gestalt Psychology,* Harcourt, Brace, New York, 1938, pp. 300-314.

Zeller, A. F. An experimental analogue of repression: I. Historical summary. *Psychological Bulletin* **47,** 39-51 (1950a).

Zeller, A. F. An experimental analogue of repression: II. The effect of individual failure and success on memory measured by relearning. *Journal of Experimental Psychology* **40,** 441-442 (1950b).

Zeller, A. F. An experimental analogue of repression: III. The effect of induced failure and success on memory measured by recall. *Journal of Experimental Psychology* **42,** 32-38 (1952).

Index